EXCLUSION OF SOCIAL SERIES AND SEXUAL MINORITIES

ELIO E

ELIO ENDLESS PUBLISHERS

Copyright © 2022 By Elio Endless. All rights reserved. No part of this book may be used or reproduced in any form whatsoever without written permission except in the case of brief quotations in critical articles or reviews. Printed in the United States of America.

For more information or to book an event, please contact: elioendleeshouse@gmail.com

Book design by Kai

Cover design by Tyson

Paperback ISBN:

ebook ISBN:

To Dad, Mom, and my supportive colleagues,Your love, guidance, and unwavering support have been the driving force behind my journey as a writer. Thank you for believing in me and encouraging me to pursue my dreams. Your presence in my life has made all the difference.

With heartfelt gratitude,

ELIO.E

Preface

Hey there, "wave"! How's it going? I'm your friendly neighborhood book editor, here to tell you about this amazing book that just landed on our shelves. It's a gem that our awesome publishing company has brought to life. Now, as part of my job, I get to dive into countless books, and I must say, this one is an absolute delight. No need for any unnecessary delay, let me give you a sneak peek into what makes it so worthwhile. Are you ready? Let's jump right in with the introduction. To be designated a sexual minority, a group's members must have a sexual identity, orientation, or practices that are not shared by the majority of the population. Most often, it refers to those who identify as lesbian, gay, bisexual, or non-heterosexual, but it can also be used to describe people who do not identify with either the male or female genders or who are transgender, non-binary (including third gender[4]), or intersex. The acronyms GSM (for "Gender and Sexual Minorities"), GSRM (for "Gender, Sexual, and Romantic Minorities"), and GSD (for "Gender and Sexual Diversity") are all variations.[8] In spite of the fact that these issues have been debated in academia, the "Sexual and Gender Minority" category has made the most headway since 2014.[9] It was announced in 2015 that the National Institutes of Health (NIH) would establish the Sexual and Gender Minority Research Office. Many different academic and professional groups have adopted the phrase since then. The term "sexual and gender minority" is broad enough to embrace not only people who identify as "LGBTI" (which stands for "lesbian, gay, bisexual, transgender, and intersex") but also people whose sexual orientation or gender identity is not binary. Queer, questioning, two-spirit, asexual, men who have sex with other men, and gender variant people are included, as are people with medical conditions that affect reproductive development (such as people with differences or disorders of sex development, who may sometimes identify as intersex).

The book The Erotic Minorities: A Swedish View by Lars Ullerstam, published in the late 1960s, popularized the term "sexual minority" by advocating for greater understanding and acceptance of individuals with paraphilias like pedophilia and other sexual orientations that were once stigmatized as "sex criminals." The phrase "sexual minority" owes much of its origin and meaning to this book.[16] This expression was used in a way that could be compared to a marginalized group. The term is supported by scientists like Ritch Savin-Williams because it helps them describe young people who don't fit into the categories of commonly used culturally defined sexual identity labels (lesbian, gay, bisexual, etc.), but who still feel attracted to people of the same anatomical sex. The word is used to characterize adolescents who do not readily identify with any of the culturally accepted sexual orientations. Both individual and societal health issues are of concernPhysical and mental health issues may develop as a result of stress over one's social life, especially among young people. It has been found that the stigmas faced by members of sexual minorities lead to increased levels of stress. Increased coping control and social and cognitive processes raise the likelihood of psychopathology as a result of stigma-related stress.[20] Sexual minorities are subjected to a lifetime of stigma-related stress, including but not limited to homophobia, rejection, and discrimination. This leads many people to resort to concealing their true identity. The majority of respondents (80%) reported being the target of harassment in this study.[21] In addition to increasing the chance of substance abuse, exposure to such traumatic events also increases the risk of developing major depressive disorder and generalized anxiety disorder.

The CDC published their 2015 research on large cohorts of ninth through twelfth grade students in the United States in 2015. One hundred different health behaviors were identified as putting LGBT youth at risk for negative health outcomes in the study. It has been found that members of sexual minorities are more likely to engage in potentially harmful behaviors than members of other minority groups. Some of the students "had no sexual contact [and] were excluded from analyses on sexual behaviors [including] female students who had sexual contact with only females [and were excluded from analyses on condom use and birth control use..." In addition, "male students who had sexual contact with only males" were excluded from studies of contraceptive use since they did not meet the criteria for exclusion.[2] In a small study, American psychologist Mark L. Hatzenbuehler found that compared to their heterosexual counterparts, LGBTQ youth were more likely to be victims of crime, to have higher rates of psychopathology, to run away from home, to use highly addictive substances, and to have multiple sexual partners. Increase and development Based on studies of adolescents, we know that the concerns and demands of sexual minorities are similar to those of their heterosexual peers. Researchers have found that sexual minority youth, particularly specifically lesbian, gay, bisexual, and transgender (LGBT) youth, are more likely to suffer emotional and physical health issues than their heterosexual peers. Epidemiology is the study of disease and its causes. Members of sexual minorities are more likely to seek out and use complementary and alternative medicine to address their particular health care needs than their heterosexual peers.[23] Sexual minority women have a higher prevalence of asthma, obesity, arthritis, and cardiovascular disease than do women from other groups. Adolescents who identify as members of sexual minorities report a higher incidence of the following compared to their heterosexual classmates: feeling unsafe on their way to or while at school, and deciding not to attend as a result.someone they were seeing or going out with forced them to do something sexual they

Acknowledgements

I would like to take this opportunity to extend my heartfelt thanks to all the individuals who have played a significant role in the creation of this non-fiction book. Your unwavering support, valuable advice, and constant encouragement have been invaluable throughout this journey. I am deeply grateful to those who have provided me with aspirational direction, constructive criticism, and kind advice. Your feedback has been instrumental in shaping the content and direction of this book. I genuinely appreciate your candid insights into my project.I am particularly grateful for the exceptional assistance of Mr. Jaffer and Mrs. Sameena at Endless Publishers. Their continuous support, dedication, and guidance have been instrumental in helping me overcome obstacles and improve the quality of my work. I am sincerely appreciative of their tremendous efforts and unwavering belief in this project.I would also like to express my heartfelt appreciation to Mr. Ahmed, my project's external advisor from Ahmed Corporation. His invaluable advice, insightful critique, and vast wisdom have played a pivotal role in refining my thoughts and enhancing the overall quality of this book. I am truly grateful for his guidance and exper tise. Furthermore, I would like to acknowledge Ms. Sultana and every individual who has contributed to obtaining the necessary resources and making this initiative possible. Your assistance, whether it was in sourcing information, conducting research, or providing logistical support, is deeply appreciated. This book would not have come to fruition without your invaluable contributions. I cannot overlook the individual who initially sparked the flame of inspiration within me to embark on this book-writing endeavor. Your unwavering belief in my abilities, continuous motivation, and unending support throughout this artistic process have been instrumental in my journey. I am forever indebted to you for being my constant source of inspiration. I want to express my deepest gratitude to every person who has contributed to this project, no matter how small their role may have been. Each and every one of you has played a part in making this book possible, and your contributions have not gone unnoticed. Your support, encouragement, and assistance have been instrumental in bringing this book to fruition. Finally, I would like to give special credit to Kai, B.EE, and Tyson, the pen names that have accompanied me on this writing adventure. Your creativity, distinct perspectives, and unique insights have added depth and character to this book. I am honored to have had the opportunity to collaborate with you. To all of you who have been a part of this remarkable journey, I extend my deepest gratitude. Your unwavering support, guidance, and friendship have been invaluable. Thank you for believing in me and for contributing to the realization of this non-fiction book. With

sincere appreciation,

Elio Endless

EDITOR NOTE

1. Publisher Notes: This edition is a product of inspiration from other works, with a portion of its content derived from public domain sources. Elioendless, the creator, editor, and publisher of the ebook edition, utilized manuscripts, select texts, and illustrative images from public domain archives. Members can acquire this ebook from our website for personal use. However, please note that any form of commercial storage, transmission, or reverse engineering of this file is strictly prohibited.

Contents

	XXIII
1. Sexual minority	1

   The beginnings

   The strain

   Acts fraught with danger

   Growth and progress

   The study of epidemiology

   There was discrimination.

   In various forms of media.

   Concerns rooted in culture

   Conflict of opinion

   The Social Network

   The making of something

   A casting

   Creating a movie

   The manufacture of rowing

   The Social Network music is the topic of this essay.

   Promotional Attempts.

Theatrical Previews

Set you free

Take home pay

Reaction from the critics

Personal media devices

The primary page is a list of the awards that have been bestowed for The Social Network.

Accuracy in historical research

Initial indications of influence

Evaluation following the 2010s

The potential continuation

Understanding Sexual Minorities is the First Step.

The Gender Enigma or Paradox.

Research dealing with gender identity in its many forms.

History of Sexual Minorities in India.

2. Sexology   67

    Early on

    After the end of WWII

    century of the 21st

    History of human sexuality

    The sources

    The Kama Sutra depicted as a painting.

    The Kama Sutra depicted as a painting.

    Fresco frescoes that were painted inside the Ajanta caves

Observation of anal sexual activity between two males.

Dynasty of the Qing

Three pages from an erotic album that was written in Chinese. Between the years 1701 and 1900?

A work of art. This is Wang Sheng. Before the year 1645

The primary article on the subject of sexuality in Japan

Greco-Roman antiquity

It was Oinochoe. The artist known as Shuvalov. In the vicinity of 430–420 BCE

The region of Etruria

Polynésie française

Yuri Lisyansky, from his autobiography

The 20th century: the shift in sexual mores

Jewish religion

The Christian faith

Islam (faith)

Religions based on Dharma

Both sex and technology

The zoophobia

Sexual exploitation

Diseases that are transmitted by sexual contacts transmitted sexually and safe sexual practices

AIDS

3. health requirements   119
    The Existing Knowledge Gap
    The Final Thoughts.

Summary   193

Chapter   209

Conclusion   210

One

Sexual minority

A group that is considered to be a sexual minority is one that has a sexual identity, orientation, or practices that are distinct from those of the majority of the society around them. It is most commonly used to refer to those who are lesbian, gay, bisexual, or non-heterosexual; however, it can also be used to refer to individuals who are transgender, non-binary (including third gender[4]), or intersex. Variants include GSM (which stands for "Gender and Sexual Minorities"), GSRM ("Gender, Sexual and Romantic Minorities"), and GSD (which stands for "Gender and Sexual Diversity").[8] Although they have been discussed in academic circles, [a] the "Sexual and Gender Minority" category has made the most progress since 2014.[9] The National Institutes of Health (NIH) made the announcement in 2015 that it will be forming the Sexual and Gender Minority Research Office. Since then, a wide variety of professional and academic organizations have used the phrase. The term "sexual and gender minority" is an umbrella word that incorporates both populations that are included in the abbreviation "LGBTI" (which stands for "lesbian, gay, bisexual, transgender, and intersex") as well as those whose sexual orientation or gender identity varies. It includes people who might not consider themselves to be part of the LGBTI community (for example, queer, questioning, two-spirit, asexual, men who have sex with other men, gender variant), as well as people who have a specific medical condition that affects reproductive development (for example, individuals with differences or disorders of sex development, who might sometimes identify as intersex).

The beginnings

The term "sexual minority" was most likely coined in the late 1960s under the influence of Lars Ullerstam's book The Erotic Minorities: A Swedish View, which is strongly in favor of tolerance and empathy to paraphilias such as pedophilia and uncommon sexualities in which people were labeled "sex criminals." This book was the most significant factor in the development of the term "sexual minority."[16] This phrase was employed in a manner comparable to that of an ethnic minority. Scientists such as Ritch Savin-Williams support the use of the term in order to accurately describe adolescent youths who may not identify as any common culturally defined sexual identity label (lesbian, gay, bisexual, etc.), but who still have attractions towards those of the same anatomical sex as themselves. The purpose of using the term is to accurately describe adolescent youths who may not identify as any common culturally defined sexual identity label. Concerns related to both people's health and their communities

The strain

Especially with young people, problems with one's physical and mental health might be a consequence of social concerns. It has been discovered that members of sexual minorities are subjected to higher levels of stress as a result of stigmas. This stress, which is associated to stigma, results in increased coping regulation as well as social and cognitive processes, which increases the risk of psychopathology.[20] Homophobia, rejection, and discrimination are just a few examples of the types of stigma-related stress that sexual minorities are forced to endure throughout their lives. As a result, many individuals are forced to hide their identities. According to the findings of the research, around eighty percent of these people claimed that they had been harassed.[21] The exposure to these kinds of traumatic events raises the individual's risk of developing major depressive disorder and generalized anxiety disorder, in addition to raising the individual's likelihood of abusing substances like alcohol and narcotics.

Acts fraught with danger

The Centers for Disease Control and Prevention (CDC) published their study from 2015 in 2015 of large cohorts of ninth to twelfth grade students across the United States. The study found that 100 health behaviors put LGBT kids at risk for adverse health consequences. those who identify as a sexual minority are more likely to participate in risky behaviors than those who identify as a nonsexual minority. Some of the students "had no sexual contact [and] were excluded from analyses on sexual behaviors [including] female students who had sexual contact with only females [and] were excluded from analyses on condom use and birth control use…" "Male students who had sexual contact with only males" were also removed from the analyses conducted on birth control use because they did not qualify as "male students who had sexual contact with only males."[2] One small study that was carried out by an American psychologist by the name of Mark L. Hatzenbuehler revealed that homosexual, bisexual, transgender, and queer (LGBTQ) adolescents were more likely to be victims of crime, had higher rates of psychopathology, were more likely to run away from home, were more likely to use highly addictive substances, and were more likely to have multiple sexual partners than heterosexual adolescents.

Growth and progress

It has been determined, on the basis of research conducted on teenagers, that the developmental needs and concerns of sexual minorities are comparable to those of heterosexual adolescents. On the other hand, studies have shown that young people who belong to sexual minorities, and more especially LGBT youth, are more likely to experience mental and physical health problems than heterosexual adolescents.

The study of epidemiology

To a greater extent than their heterosexual counterparts, members of sexual minorities are more likely to seek out and make use of alternative and complementary medicine in order to meet their personal health care requirements.[23] Women who are members of sexual minorities are more likely to suffer from asthma, obesity, arthritis, and cardiovascular illness than women who are members of other groups. When compared to heterosexual pupils, adolescents who identify as members of sexual minorities report a higher incidence of the following: having the impression that they are not safe when traveling to and from school or while attending school and choosing not to go to school because they have this impression.being forced to engage in sexual activity that they did not want to do by someone they were seeing or going out with at least once throughout the course of the previous year (such as being forced to touch, kiss, or engage in sexual activity physically). having sexual activity, having one's first sexual experience before the age of 13, having sexual activity with at least four other persons who were not using birth control, and having a history of sexual abuse are all risk factors for having sexual activity.Sexual minorities are at a higher risk for self-inflicted harm when compared to the general population as a whole.[25] It appears that ageism has a larger role in determining how older members of sexual minorities are treated. It would appear that support for aging members of sexual minorities is widespread.[26]

There was discrimination.

Adults who identified as gay, lesbian, or bisexual were more likely to report being discriminated against than adults who identified with any other sexual orientation. This discrimination was found to have a favorable association with both detrimental impacts on quality of life as well as indications of psychiatric morbidity.[27] In addition, in comparison to those who identified as heterosexual, those who identified as bisexual or homosexual were more likely to report having one of the five psychiatric illnesses that were investigated.[27] It was clear that the hostility and prejudice that these homosexual individuals were subjected to had a negative effect on them, which led to alterations in their mental state.

In various forms of media.

The majority of the time, the portrayal of sexual minorities in mainstream media is one of being disregarded, trivialized, or reviled. Their lack of categorization can be explained by the term "symbolic annihilation," which arises from the fact that they do not conform to the white, heterosexual, vanilla sort of lifestyle. It has been hypothesized that the realm of internet media has evolved into a place where members of sexual minorities are able to employ "social artillery." This explanation focuses on how individuals might combat homophobia through the use of social networking and interactions with other individuals.[28] However, there are some people who have broken into the public eye through the mediums of television and music. Several popular television programs, including "The Ellen DeGeneres Show" and "Modern Family," have cast members who aren't afraid to be upfront about their sexual orientations other than heterosexuality. People in the music industry like as Sam Smith and Sia have achieved success with songs that convey their feelings and sexuality and have a large number of fans. Even if sexual minorities do have a place in the media, it is a common criticism that their representations are still very limited. In television series, a character who is gay is frequently a one-dimensional caricature who serves no purpose other than to provide comedic relief or a twist to the story. In contrast to their heteronormative counterparts, members of the sexual minority are frequently relegated to supporting roles. On the other hand, ever since non-heterosexual performers, musicians, and characters have been integrated into mainstream media, the concept of non-normativity has been more acceptable in contemporary society.[29]

Concerns rooted in culture

The research that has been done in the recent past as well as the current one is "skewed toward SM men—and is disproportionately focused on HIV and other sexually transmitted infections." Between the years 1989 and 2011, the National Institutes of Health (NIH) in the United States sponsored and supported a large number of grants for research, however funded research on sexual minorities and health only made up 0.1% of all funded studies. The majority of study has been conducted on males who identify as gay or bisexual. The percentage of women and sexual minorities studying was 13.5%. When compared to people in other nations, sexual minorities in South Africa have health disparities that are directly tied to their sexual orientation. South Africa is home to one of the highest rates of reported sexual assaults committed against women who identify with a sexual minority. Particularly at risk are women of color who are already residing in urban areas with low incomes. The perpetrators of sexual violence feel that they are "correcting the women" and that their actions would cure the victims of their homosexuality. They also believe that they are "making the women straight."

Conflict of opinion

For the purposes of verification, this section needs further citations. Please assist in the improvement of this article by adding citations to sources that can be relied upon in this particular area. Content that lacks appropriate citations may be contested and removed. March of

2017 (Find out how and when this message can be removed from templates)The vast majority of persons who identify as LGBT take issue with the term "sexual minorities" and instead prefer the term "LGBTQ." There may be a variety of reasons behind these complaints. People who identify as lesbian, gay, bisexual, transgender, or queer (LGBTQ) may feel that the term "sexual minority" brings up memories of being subjected to discrimination and of their status as a minority. They do not wish to be regarded as a separate minority but rather as an important and respected member of the larger society. People who identify as BDSM, swingers, polyamorists, and other "sexual strangers" are among those who reject the phrase because it is too inclusive. In other words, they want to make it abundantly apparent that these sexual behaviors are not the same thing as bisexuality, homosexuality, or transgender identity in order to prevent confusion. Other factors contribute to the distaste that some transgender and transsexual people have for the term "sexual minority." They contend that the phenomenon of transsexuality or transgender identity has nothing to do with sex, sexual behaviors, or sexual orientation; rather, they assert that it is related to gender, gender dysphoria, and gender-variant behavior or feelings. Because of this, they believe that it is inaccurate to categorize them as a "sexual minority," given that they are, in fact, a gender-variant minority. The opposition of some conservative groups to the use of the phrase "sexual minority" stems from an entirely separate set of concerns.

They believe or have the impression that the term naturally implies some degree of legalization or protection for people engaging in such sexual acts. This is comparable to the way in which members of ethnic minorities are protected from being discriminated against or prosecuted in modern democratic countries. The majority of people have a negative opinion of the term because it contains the word "minority." Additionally, they contend that not all of these categories are entirely about minorities but rather about groups that are considered to be minorities. Others who are considered to be members of "sexual minorities" include fetishists and those who participate in BDSM (bondage, domination, and submission), as well as sadists and masochists.[19] A sexuals, ficto sexuals, and those whose choice of partner or partners is unconventional, such as swingers, polyamorists, or people in other non-monogamous relationships, as well as people who have partners who are much older or younger than themselves, may also fall under this category.[36] It may also refer to those who are involved in a relationship with someone of a different race.

Typically, the phrase "sexual minority" is exclusively applied to groups that engage in sexual activity on the basis of mutual consent: For instance, it is not common to refer to people who commit rape as members of a sexual minority. However, the word can be used to refer to anyone whose sexuality plays a significant and fetishized role in the act of voluntarily acting out a rape fantasy. Also, someone who occasionally mixes consensual kink[35] or same-sex action into their otherwise heterosexual sex life is not typically considered to be a member of a sexual minority.

The Social Network

The Accidental Billionaires by Ben Mezrich served as the inspiration for the biographical drama film The Social Network, which was released in the United States in 2010 and was directed by David Fincher and scripted by Aaron Sorkin. It tells the story of how the social networking website Facebook got its start. Jesse Eisenberg plays Mark Zuckerberg, the founder of Facebook, while Andrew Garfield plays Eduardo Saverin, Justin Timberlake plays Sean Parker, Armie Hammer plays Cameron and Tyler Winklevoss, and Max Minghella plays Divya Narendra. Justin Timberlake also plays Sean Parker. Although Saverin served as a consultant for Mezrich's book, neither Mark Zuckerberg nor any other member of the Facebook crew was involved in the project in any way.

When Sorkin agreed to write the script, production officially got under way. The principal photography began in October of that same year in Cambridge, Massachusetts, and continued through November of that same year. Additional sequences were filmed in the state of California, specifically in the cities of Pasadena and Los Angeles. Trent Reznor and Atticus Ross of Nine Inch Nails composed the score for the film, which was released on September 28, 2010. The score won an award for its excellence.

The film had its world premiere at the New York Film Festival on September 24, 2010, and Sony Pictures Releasing opened it in theaters across the United States on October 1. The movie was a huge success both critically and commercially, bringing in $224 million on a budget of only $40 million, and receiving praise from a wide variety of reviewers. 78 critics chose it as one of the best films of the year, and 22 critics chose it as the finest film of the year; this was the most critics that chose the best film of any film that year. In addition to that, the National Board of Review deemed it to be the finest movie of the year 2010. It garnered eight nominations at the 83rd Academy Awards, including for Best Picture, Best Director, and Best Actor for Eisenberg, and it won for Best Adapted Screenplay, Best Original Score, and Best Film Editing. Eisenberg also took home the award for Best Actor in the film. At the 68th annual Golden Globe honors, it also won honors for Best Motion Picture – Drama, Best Director, Best Screenplay, and Best Original Score. The Social Network has maintained a strong reputation since its initial release, and it is commonly cited by critics as one of the best films of the 2010s and 21st century. [5][6][7][8] The Writers Guild of America ranked Sorkin's screenplay the third greatest of the 21st century. [9] Although there has been no official announcement regarding a sequel, Sorkin has publicly expressed interest and willingness to write a screenplay for one should Fincher return

Plot

Mark Zuckerberg, then 19 years old and a student at Harvard University, learns on October 28, 2003 that his girlfriend, Erica Albright, has broken up with him. When Zuckerberg got back to his hostel, he immediately started writing a derogatory post about Albright on his LiveJournal blog. After hacking into college databases to obtain images of female students, he establishes a campus website called Facemash and allows visitors to the site to score the attractiveness of the students shown in the photos. Zuckerberg is placed on academic probation for a period of six months after the traffic to the website brought down parts of the computer network at Harvard. However, the twins Cameron and Tyler Winklevoss, together with their business partner Divya Narendra, became interested in Facemash as a result of its success. The three individuals extend an invitation to Zuckerberg to participate in the development of Harvard Connection, a social network that is restricted to Harvard students and focuses on dating. Zuckerberg approaches his buddy Eduardo Saverin with the concept for Thefacebook, a social networking website that would only be accessible to students enrolled in Ivy League universities. Saverin supplies Zuckerberg with initial financing in the amount of $1,000, which enables the latter to create the website, which immediately gains a large following. When the Winklevoss twins and Narendra discover about Thefacebook, they are enraged because they believe that Zuckerberg stole their idea while also deceiving them by pausing development on the Harvard Connection website. They take their protest to Larry Summers, the President of Harvard University, but he is unconcerned and believes that disciplinary action against TheFacebook or Zuckerberg would serve little use. Christy Lee, a fellow student, introduces herself to Saverin and Zuckerberg and asks them to "Facebook me," a phrase that leaves an impression on them. As TheFacebook's user base continues to swell, Zuckerberg decides to extend the reach of the network to include Yale University, Columbia University, and Stanford University. Saverin and Zuckerberg are introduced to Napster co-founder Sean Parker, who describes his "billion-dollar" ambition for the company. Lee is the one who makes the introductions. Saverin thinks Zuckerberg is insane and paranoid, but Zuckerberg is impressed by what he sees. Additionally, Parker advises changing the name of the website to Facebook. Later on, on Parker's recommendation, Zuckerberg moves the company to Palo Alto, while Saverin stays in New York to continue working on the company's business development. Parker subsequently moves into the house that Zuckerberg is using as a base of operations and becomes more involved with the company, much to Saverin's anger. Zuckerberg is utilizing the property as a base of operations.

While competing for Harvard against the Hollandia Roeiclub in the Henley Royal Regatta in 2004, the Winklevoss twins found out that Facebook had extended to Europe with Oxford, Cambridge, and LSE. They made the decision to sue the corporation for intellectual property theft as a result of this discovery. In the meantime, Saverin opposes to Parker making business choices for Facebook, which leads to a fight that results in the freezing of the company's bank account. When Zuckerberg discloses that they have acquired $500,000 from angel investor Peter Thiel, it is enough to convince him to change his mind. When Saverin learns that the new investment deal will allow his portion of Facebook to be reduced from 34% to 0.03% while maintaining the ownership percentages of all other parties, he becomes outraged. Before being kicked out of the building, he has a confrontation with Zuckerberg and Parker, during which Saverin makes a promise to sue Zuckerberg. Saverin's name has been deleted from the company's masthead, where it previously appeared as the co-founder and CFO. In later events, Parker gets arrested for possessing cocaine while attending a party to celebrate one million users. Because of his attempt to place blame on Saverin, Zuckerberg severed all relations with him and told him to go home. The Winklevoss twins have claimed in separate depositions that Zuckerberg stole their idea, while Saverin has claimed that his shares of Facebook were unfairly diluted when the firm was founded. Both of these claims have been made public. Marylin Delpy, a young lawyer for the defense, tells Mark Zuckerberg that they will settle with Eduardo Saverin because the sordid aspects of Facebook's founding and Zuckerberg's heartless attitude will make a jury unable to empathize with Zuckerberg.

While by himself, Zuckerberg sends a friend request to Albright on Facebook and keeps refreshing the screen to see whether she accepts.

- Cast

- Mark Zuckerberg portrayed by Jesse Eisenberg

- [12] Andrew Garfield plays the role of Eduardo Saverin.

- [13] Justin Timberlake in the role of Sean Parker

- Cameron and Tyler Winklevoss are played by Armie Hammer

- [14] Max Minghella in the role of Divya Narendra

- Christy Lee portrayed by Brenda Song

- Marylin Delpy portrayed by Rashida Jones

- John Getz in the role of Sy

- David Selby plays the role of Gage

- Gretchen was played by Denise Grayson (position

- [17] Douglas Urbanski in the role of Larry Summers

- Erica Albright portrayed by Rooney Mara

- Dustin Moskovitz is portrayed here by Joseph Mazzello

- The election of Dustin Fitzsimons as President of The Phoenix – Sk Club

- Peter Thiel portrayed by Wallace Langham

- [14] Patrick Mapel in the role of Chris Hughes

- Amelia Ritter is portrayed here by Dakota Johnson

- Alice Cantwel portrayed by Malese Jow

- Trevor Wright plays the role of B.U. [17] A man wearing a bra

- Shelby Young as King of the Champions

- [17] Aaron Sorkin in the Role of an Advertising Executive

- Bill Gates, portrayed by Steve Sires

- Caleb Landry Jones during his time as a member of the fraternity

Hammer is portrayed by Josh Pence, whose body is digitally altered to seem like Hammer. Hammer's likeness was digitally overlaid onto Pence's body. In the film's closing credits, he is credited with Hammer as performing the role of Tyler Winklevoss. In addition, he has a cameo appearance in which he plays the part of a man who Zuckerberg and Saverin divert from going to the bathroom. [24]

The making of something

In an interview, screenwriter Aaron Sorkin stated, "What attracted me to [the film project] had nothing to do with Facebook. The invention itself is as modern as it gets, but the story is as old as storytelling; the themes of friendship, loyalty, jealousy, class, and power." Sorkin went on to say that he read an unfinished draft of The Accidental Billionaires when the publisher began "shopping it around" for a film adaptation. Sorkin continued by saying, "I was reading it, and somewhere on page three I said yes. It was the fastest I said yes to anything. They wanted me to start right away. Ben and I were kind of doing our research at the same time, sort of along parallel lines." Sorkin claims that Mezrich did not send him excerpts from his book as he was writing it: "Two or three times we'd get together. I'd go to Boston, or we'd meet in New York and kind of compare notes and share information, but I didn't see the book until he was done with it. By the time I saw the book, I was probably 80 percent done with the screenplay." [25] Sorkin elaborated: "Two or three times we There is a lot of information that is available, and in addition to that, I conducted a lot of research in the first person with a number of the people who were engaged in the tale. Because most of the people who did it did so on the condition of anonymity, I can't go into too much detail about it, but what I did find was that two lawsuits were brought against Facebook at roughly the same time, that the defendant, plaintiffs, and witnesses all came into a deposition room and swore under oath, and that three different versions of the story were told. I opted to exaggerate the idea that there were three different versions of the narrative being told rather than choosing one and determining that it is the most truthful version or choosing one and deciding that it is the most juicy version of the story. That's how I came up with the layout of the room where the deposition would take place [25].

A casting

Casting began in the middle of 2009, with Jesse Eisenberg, Justin Timberlake, and Andrew Garfield announced to star. [26][27] Jonah Hill was in contention for Timberlake's role, but director David Fincher passed on him. [28] In October 2009, Brenda Song, Rooney Mara, Armie Hammer, Shelby Young, and Josh Pence were cast. [29] Max Minghella and Dakota Johnson were also confirmed. [29] Eisenberg stated in an interview with The Baltimore Sun that

Creating a movie

Principal photography began in October 2009 in Cambridge, Massachusetts.[31] Scenes were filmed around the campuses of two Massachusetts prep schools, Phillips Academy and Milton Academy.[32] Additional scenes were filmed on the campus of Wheelock College, which was set up to be Harvard's campus.[33] (Harvard has turned down most requests for on-location filming ever since the filming of Love Story (1970), which caused significant physical damage to trees on campus.)[34] Filming took place on the Keyser and Wyman quadrangles in the Homewood campus of Johns Hopkins University from November 2–4,[35] which also doubled for Harvard in the film.[36] The first scene in the film, where Zuckerberg is with his girlfriend, took 99 takes to finish.[4] The film was shot on the Red One digital cinema camera.[37] The rowing scenes with the Winklevoss brothers were filmed at Community Rowing Inc. in Newton, Massachusetts[38] and at the Henley Royal Regatta; miniature faking process was used in a sequence showing a rowing event at the latter.[39] Although a significant portion of the latter half of the film is set in Silicon Valley, the filmmakers opted to shoot those scenes in Los Angeles and Pasadena.

During the filming of the moments in which Armie Hammer was cast as one of the Winklevoss twins, Josh Pence served as his stand-in and assisted him in performing his lines. In post-production, his face was eventually digitally grafted onto Pence's face, and in other situations, split-screen shooting was used. Pence was apprehensive about not having much face time during the job, but after much deliberation, he thought of the part as a "no-brainer" Hammer states that director David Fincher "likes to push himself and likes to push technology" and is "one of the most technologically minded guys I've ever met."[40] This included sending the actors to "twin boot camp" for 10 months to learn everything about the Winklevosses. [24] Hammer states that director David Fincher "likes to push himself and likes to push technology" and is "one of the most technologically minded guys I've ever met."

The manufacture of rowing

The film depicts the long-standing rowing tradition at Harvard University. Community Rowing Inc. held a casting call and a tryout for 20 rowing extras; some of the participants were graduates from Harvard, Northeastern University, Boston University, George Washington University, and Trinity College, as well as local club rowers from Union Boat Club and Riverside Boat Club. [41] None of the cast rowing extras for the Henley Royal Regatta racing scene appeared in the film; filming for the race was originally planned to take place in Los Angeles, but director David Fincher decided to move it Dawn Reagan, a coach from Loyola Marymount, was engaged by David Fincher to assist in the training of Josh Pence and Armie Hammer. [43] While Hammer was new to the discipline of rowing, Pence had previous experience rowing while attending Dartmouth College. The indoor rowing scene was captured on camera at the indoor rowing tanks at Boston University. During filming, every single one of Boston University's (BU) blue oars was given a coat of Harvard's crimson paint. [42] Dan Boyne served as the official rowing consultant for both the United States and the United Kingdom.

The Social Network music is the topic of this essay.

It was announced on June 1, 2010, that Trent Reznor and Atticus Ross would be scoring the film. [44] The soundtrack was released on September 28, in various formats under the Null Corporation label. [45] Leading up to the release of the soundtrack, a free five-track EP was made available for download. [46] The White Stripes' song "Ball and Biscuit" can be heard in the opening of the film, and The Beatles' song "Baby, You're a Rich Man" Neither song is included on the album that serves as the soundtrack. Both the Golden Globe Award for Best Original Score in 2011 and the Academy Award for Best Original Score in 2011 went to Trent Reznor and Atticus Ross for their work on "The Social Network."

Promotional Attempts.

As Neil Kellerhouse had previously designed posters for the films of Steven Soderbergh, a friend of director David Fincher's, he was contacted by Ceán Chaffin in late 2009 to work on the key art for The Social Network, which had to make sole use of one approved photograph, that of Eisenberg's head. The first theatrical poster, designed by Neil Kellerhouse, was released on June 18, 2010. [48] As Keaton wanted to highlight the tremendous drama that went along with Mark Zuckerberg's success,

Theatrical Previews

The film's first teaser trailer was released on June 25, 2010.[52] The second teaser was released on July 8.[53] The full length theatrical trailer debuted on July 16, 2010, which plays an edited version of the song "Creep", originally by Radiohead, covered by the Belgian choir group Scala & Kolacny Brothers.[54][55] The trailer was then shown in theaters, prior to the films Inception, Dinner for Schmucks, Salt, Easy A, The Virginity Hit, and The Other Guys. Mark Woollen & Associates was responsible for the production of the theatrical trailer, which went on to win the Grand Key Art prize at the 2011 Key Art Awards[56], which were hosted by The Hollywood Reporter. In addition, the trailer was included on The Film Informant's list of the Perfect 10 Trailers in 2010.[57]

Set you free

On September 24, 2010, at the New York Film Festival, a screening of The Social Network was presented for the very first time. [1]

Take home pay

During the weekend of October 1-3, 2010, the movie was made available to watch in cinemas around the United States. It broke Inception's record for the smallest second weekend drop for any number-one film of 2010, with a drop of only 31.2%. [3] The film maintained the top spot in its second weekend, grossing $22.4 million in 2,771 theaters. [3] It was the third-smallest drop overall, behind Secretariat's 25.1% drop and Tooth Fairy's 28.6% drop. [3] It broke Inception's record. Following the conclusion of its run in theaters, the movie earned a total of $224.9 million worldwide, including $97 million in the United States of America and $128 million in other markets. [3]

Reaction from the critics

At the 2010 New York Film Festival are, from left to right, Aaron Sorkin, Jesse Eisenberg, Andrew Garfield, and Justin Timberlake. David Fincher is in the far rightmost position. On the website Rotten Tomatoes, the movie has had 326 reviews and has received an approval rating of 96%, which is equivalent to an average rating of 9 out of 10. The website's critical consensus reads, "Impeccably scripted, beautifully directed, and filled with fine performances, The Social Network is a riveting, ambitious example of modern filmmaking at its finest." [58] On Metacritic, the film has a weighted average score of 95 out of 100, based on 42 critics, indicating "universal acclaim". [59] Audiences polled by CinemaScore gave the film an average grade of "B+" Peter Bradshaw from The Guardian gave the film four stars and praised David Fincher's directing as having the "right intensity and claustrophobia for a story that takes place largely in a stupefyingly male environment at Harvard University in 2003".[61] Kaitlyn Tiffany from The Verge wrote positive comments on Aaron Sorkin's screenplay, writing that his "reflex for writing witty, whiny men with outsized intellect and poorly disguised narcissis

Roger Ebert of the Chicago Sun-Times awarded it four stars and named it the best film of the year. He wrote: "David Fincher's film has the rare quality of not only being as smart as its brilliant hero, but in the same way. It is cocksure, impatient, cold, exciting and instinctively perceptive." [66] Peter Travers of Rolling Stone awarded the film his first full four-star rating of the year and said: "The Social Network is the movie of the year "The biographical part takes liberties with its subject. Aaron Sorkin based his screenplay on [...] The Accidental Billionaires, so everything that's seen isn't necessarily to be believed," wrote Joe Morgenstern in The Wall Street Journal. [69] Among the film's very few negative reviewers was Nathan Heller of Slate, who described it as "rote and deeply mediocre" as well as "maddeningly generic," and believed that, "Sorkin and Fincher's collaboration According to an aggregation done by Metacritic, The Social Network made it onto the top-ten rankings of the greatest films of 2010 compiled by 78 different cinema critics. The film received first place rankings from 22 of the critics, while it received second place rankings from 12 of the critics. The Social Network was the film that was featured on the most top-ten lists for 2010. [71][72] In 2016, the BBC announced that the film had been ranked as the 27th-best film of the 21st century by 177 film reviewers from around the world. [73] The script was ranked as the fourth best American screenplay of the 21st century by writers for IndieWire in 2018. Michael Nordine argued that "everything came together nearly perfectly on the film, thanks in large part to Aaron Sorkin's Oscar-winning screenplay. Its finds the loquacious scribe at his best, with all of the verbal takedowns [...] and rapid-fire back-and-forths we've come to expect (and, more often than not, love) from

Personal media devices

On January 11, 2011, The Social Network was made available to purchase on DVD and Blu-ray. The DVD contains an audio commentary with director David Fincher, as well as a second discussion with writer Aaron Sorkin and the cast. Sales of the DVD totaled $13,470,305 in its first week of release, making it the most popularly purchased DVD of the week. [75] The DVD also includes a cast and crew commentary. The commentary are included on the Blu-ray and two-disc DVD editions. Additionally, a feature-length documentary titled "How Did They Ever Make a Movie of Facebook?" is included on both formats., featurettes, Angus Wall, Kirk Baxter, and Ren Klyce on Post, Trent Reznor, Atticus Ross, and David Fincher on the

Score, In the Hall of the Mountain King: Reznor's First Draft, Swarmatron, Jeff Cronenweth, and David Fincher on the Visuals, and a Ruby Skye VIP Room: Multi-Angle Scene Breakdown feature. [76] Also included is a feature titled Ruby Skye VIP Room: Multi A new Dolby Atmos mix and an upscaled Dolby Vision/HDR10 transfer from the film's 2K master were included in the film's release on Ultra HD Blu-ray in October 2021, which was a part of the Columbia Classics 4K Ultra HD Collection (Volume 2) from Columbia Home Entertainment. Honors and accolades

The primary page is a list of the awards that have been bestowed for The Social Network.

At the 68th Annual Golden Globe Awards, which were held on January 16, 2011, The Social Network took home the Golden Globe for Best Motion Picture – Drama. [78] The film also took home the Golden Globes for Best Director, Best Screenplay, and Best Original Score, making it the film with the most victories of the evening. [79] The movie was up for seven British Academy Film Awards, including Best Film, Best Actor in a Leading Role (Jesse Eisenberg), Best Actor in a Supporting Role (Andrew Garfield), and Rising Star Award (Andrew Garfield). Jesse Eisenberg won the award for Best Actor in a Leading Role. Andrew Garfield won the award for Rising Star Award. On February 13, 2011, it received three awards: one for Best Editing, one for Best Adapted Screenplay, and one for Best Direction[80]. The Social Network was nominated for eight Academy Awards, including Best Picture, Best Actor, Best Cinematography, Best Director, Best Film Editing, Best Original Score, Best Sound Mixing, and Best Adapted Screenplay. On February 27, 2011, at the 83rd Academy Awards, it won three of those awards, including Best Adapted Screenplay, Best Original Score, and Best Film Editing. It is just the third movie in history—after Schindler's List (1993) and L.A. Film Critics Association—to win the award for Best Picture from the National Board of Review, the National Society of Film Critics, the New York Film Critics Circle, and the Los Angeles Film Critics Association. The National Board of Review gave the award. Confidential (1997)—to win all "Big Four" critical prizes, as well as the "Hollywood Ensemble Award" from the Hollywood Film prizes. [82] Additionally, the film earned "Best Picture" at the Hollywood Film Awards. [83]

Accuracy in historical research

Mark Zuckerberg, the founder of Facebook, has expressed his displeasure with the film that is being created on him and has pointed out that a significant portion of the plot of the film is not genuine. The script was discovered to be available online in July of 2009. [84][85] In November 2009, executive producer Kevin Spacey said, "The Social Network is probably going to be a lot funnier than people might expect it to be." [86] The Cardinal Courier reported that the film was about "greed, obsession, unpredictability, and sex," and it posed the question, "Despite the fact that there are over 500 million Facebook users, does this mean Facebook can become a profitable blockbuster At the D8 conference hosted by D: All Things Digital on June 2, 2010, host Kara Swisher told Zuckerberg she knew he was not happy with The Social Network being based on him, to which he replied, "I just wished that nobody made a movie of me while I was still alive." [88] Zuckerberg stated to Oprah Winfrey that the drama and partying of the film is mostly fiction, and that he had spent the majority of the previous six years focusing, working hard, and It is interesting to see my past rewritten in a way that emphasizes things that didn't matter, (like the Winklevosses, who I've still never even met and had no part in the work we did to create the site over the past 6 years), and leaves out things that really did (like the many other people in our lives at the time, who supported us in innumerable ways). This is how Facebook co-founder Dustin Moskovitz described the film. According to what Moskovitz has stated, The version presented in the trailer seems to be a lot more interesting, so I'm going to choose to recall that we drank ourselves silly and had a lot of sex with coeds. There were a lot of great things that happened in 2004, but basically we just worked a lot and freaked out about things. ... Although the storyline of the book and script unashamedly targeted Zuckerberg, I had the impression that many of his admirable traits were shown in a true manner in the trailer (with the exception of the soundtrack). At the end of the day, they are powerless to avoid portraying him as the brilliant, goal-oriented thinker that he actually is.

Eduardo Saverin, one of the company's co-founders, stated that "the movie was clearly intended to be entertainment and not a fact-based documentary." [92] Aaron Sorkin, the writer of the script, stated that "I don't want my fidelity to be to the truth; I want it to be to storytelling." [4] "Can we not have the true be the enemy of the good?" Journalist Jeff Jarvis acknowledged the film was "well-crafted," but he called it "the anti-social movie." Jarvis took issue with Sorkin's decision to change various events and characters for dramatic effect, and he dismissed the film as "the story that those who resist the change society is undergoing want to see." Technology broadcaster Leo Laporte agreed, calling the film "anti-geek and misogynistic." Sorkin responded to these allegations by saying, "I was writing about The author Andrew Clark of The Guardian wrote that "there's something insidious about this genre of [docudrama] scriptwriting," and he questioned whether or not "a 26-year-old businessman really deserves to have his name dragged through the mud in a murky mixture of fact and imagination for the general entertainment of the movie-viewing public?" Clark continued by saying, "I'm not sure whether Mark Zuckerberg is a punk, a genius, or both. But I won't be seeing The Social Network to find out." In a blog post for CNN, Pete Cashmore, founder and CEO of Mashable, said this about Facebook founder Mark Zuckerberg: "If the Facebook founder

[Zuckerberg] is concerned about being represented as anything but a genius with an industrious work ethic, he can breathe a sigh of relief." [97] Jessi Hempel, a technology writer for Fortune who claims to have known Zuckerberg "for a long time," wrote this about the film: "It's

In contrast, in the film, Zuckerberg seems more obsessed with achieving the largesse that bad boy Sean Parker, an original Napster founder, portrays when he arrives to meet Zuckerberg at a New York restaurant. [98] The real-life Zuckerberg was obsessed with creating a website that had the potential to connect everyone on the planet. [99] In the film, Zuckerberg seems more obsessed with achieving the largesse that Parker portrays. Lawrence Lessig, a professor at Harvard Law School, argued in an article published in The New Republic that Sorkin's screenplay fails to mention the "real villain" of the story:Sorkin absolutely ignores the whole and utter absurdity of a world in which entitled Harvard undergraduates' hurt feelings are adjudicated by the engines of a federal lawsuit because "our idea was stolen!" Sorkin completely ignores the complete and utter absurdity of a world in which a federal lawsuit is cranked up to arbitrate the hurt feelings of entitled Harvard undergraduates. The documentary does not provide us with sufficient information to determine whether or not there was a legitimate legal claim involved in this scenario. Sorkin has not been coy about the fact that the plot contains numerous fictitious elements; rather, he has admitted to this reality. But based on what has been shared with us, it is clear that we have sufficient information to conclude that any legal system that would sanction the behavior of these children by allowing them to blackmail the most prosperous company of this century for $65 million ought to be ashamed of itself. Has Mark Zuckerberg broken the terms of his contract? Perhaps, in which case the damages are more on the order of $650, rather than $65 million. Has he been accused of stealing a trade secret? Never in a million years. Did he steal anything else that was considered "property"? Absolutely not; he was the one who wrote the code for Facebook, and the "idea" of a social network cannot be patented in and of itself. It was not justice that resulted in the twins receiving $65 million; rather, it was the dread of a law system that was both arbitrary and inefficient. That system functions as a tax on inventiveness and originality. This tax, rather than the innovator it hampered, is the true bad guy in this scenario.

Sheryl Sandberg, the Chief Operating Officer of Facebook, stated that she had seen the movie and that it was "very Hollywood" and primarily "fiction" in the course of an onstage debate with Arianna Huffington, the co-founder of The Huffington Post, which took place in New York City during Advertising Week in 2010. She made the assertion that "in real life, he [Zuckerberg] was just sitting around with his friends in front of his computer, ordering pizza." [100] "Who wants to go see that for two hours?" Divya Narendra stated that he was "initially surprised" to see himself depicted by the non-Indian actor Max Minghella, but he also agreed that the actor did a "good job in pushing the dialogue forward and creating a sense of urgency in what was a very frustrating period" [101] Divya Narendra said that he was "initially surprised" to see himself portrayed by the non-Indian actor Max Minghella.

Initial indications of influence

Since its release, The Social Network has been cited as inspiring involvement in start-ups and social media.[102] Bob Lefsetz has stated that: "watching this movie makes you want to run from the theatre, grab your laptop and build your own empire,"[103] noting that The Social Network has helped fuel an emerging perception that "techies have become the new rock stars."[104] This has led Dave Knox to comment that: "fifteen years from now we might just look back and realize this movie inspired our next great generation of entreprene urs."[103] After seeing the movie, Zuckerberg was quoted as saying he is "interested to see what effect The Social Network has on entrepreneurship", noting that he gets "lots of messages from people who claim that they have been very much inspired... to start their own company."[105] Saverin echoed these sentiments, stating that the film may inspire "countless others to create and take that leap to start a new business."[106] In one such instance, the co-founders of Wall Street Magnate confirmed that they were inspired to create the fantasy trading community after watching The Social Network. After the success of the movie, Aaron Sorkin became attached to another project about a technology company. He wrote the script for the biopic Steve Jobs, which was released in 2015 and followed a similar structure.[108] Another film about Facebook may be produced, as Sheryl Sandberg has signed a deal with Sony Pictures Entertainment to develop her book Lean In: Women, Work, and the Will to Lead, into a movie.

Evaluation following the 2010s

After the turn of the century, critics and audiences alike agreed that The Social Network was among the top movies of the 2010s. According to Metacritic, the film was ranked on the top ten lists of over 30 different film critics for the decade of the 2010s, including eight rankings for first place and four rankings for second place. Metacritic ranked The Social Network third overall, following Mad Max: Fury Road and Moonlight.[110] Esquire named The Social Network the best of the 2010s, calling it Citizen Kane "for the Internet age" and dubbing it "the movie of our new millennium".[111] With Facebook going "from a utopian, world-shrinking force of good to a potential threat to democracy", Esquire wrote, "Fincher seemed to sense all of this and more long before anyone else. And his brilliant, troubling film bristles with that queasy sense of prophecy and prescience."[111] Polygon, calling The Social Network the best film of the decade, wrote, "The Social Network, by chance or by design, has become one of the most immensely relevant movies of this decade... But after nearly a decade of watching Facebook 'move fast and break things,' including news websites, social video, politics, etc., the movie's tangible sense of tension can easily be reinterpreted as foreboding for what comes after you make a billion friends."[112] Director Quentin Tarantino called the film the best of the 2010s, singling out the script by Aaron Sorkin, whom he described as "the greatest active dialogist".[113]

Rolling Stone ranked The Social Network second after Moonlight (2016) on its end-of-decade list, describing it as "one deliciously re-watchable preview of the apocalypse, as entertaining and cheeky as it is troubling and startlingly prescient".[114] Time Out named it the fourth-best of the decade, "Powered by a relentless, clinical Aaron Sorkin script, directed with sinuous grace by David Fincher and loaded with smirking, smart-ass central performances, The Social Network is arguably the most important and prophetic film of our era, itself a depressing thought."[115] ScreenCrush ranked The Social Network eighth, referring to it as "[Fincher's] spiritual sequel to Fight Club, another story of an embittered, lonely man who discovers unleashing his rage at society has unexpected consequences".[116] Mashable, listing The Social Network among the top 15 films of the 2010s, said of the story, "It was everything young people could be and everything older generations feared in us before a decade of blaming [us for] problems we didn't create and can't solve."[117] IndieWire ranked The Social Network sixteenth among the decade's films, writing, "The Social Network is both a thrilling, queasy exploration of how Facebook came to be and a searing indictment of what it would inevitably become."[118] Inverse listed the film among those defining "class rage" in the 2010s, "As a gently prodding diagnosis of class conflict, The Social Network is a logical place to start."

The potential continuation

In January 2019, Sorkin disclosed that Rudin has suggested the development of a screenplay for a sequel, noting that "a lot of very interesting, dramatic stuff has happened since the movie ends." [120] Sorkin also mentioned that there was indeed enough material to create a sequel. [121] On July 18, 2019, Eisenberg expressed his interests in starring in the proposed sequel, stating that "Sorkin is a genius, and if he chooses to write about something, I'll obviously be interested

Communities of people who identify as sexual minorities or third genders have established themselves in virtually every part of the world. These communities have their own regional or local identities, as well as their own traditions and practices. The narratives of a third gender regarding sexual orientation or gender identity are typically hidden from view and regarded with disdain by the majority of society. In India, there has always been a sizeable community of people who identify as belonging to sexual minorities or third genders, albeit intermittently and only in the forms that are deemed acceptable by the culture. (Such as Chakka and Hijra, amongst others) and at other times out of sight and under the radar, the concerns surrounding sexual minorities have never been given real consideration. In India, the difficulties surrounding the population of people who identify as third gender have only very recently been given thought with regard to lief. However, sexual minorities continue to be a neglected section of society. As a result, they are frequently victims of atrocities and face a variety of forms of unfair treatment or discrimination in their families, neighborhoods, communities, and throughout society as a whole. They are unable to lead a distinguished or dignified social life as a result of the varying perceptions and attitudes on them held by the larger heterosexual members and cis gender people (CIS gender: pertaining to an individual whose sense of personal identity and gender corresponds with their birth sex.) of the society. They are unable to do this because of the attitudes held by the larger heterosexual members of the society.

In today's culture, those who belong to sexual minorities are, for the most part, not accepted. The excluded groups (such as sexual minorities) are typically deprived of a means of subsistence, secured permanent employment, earnings, education, property and land ownerships, skills, democratic participation, utilization of public goods, citizenship, and legal equality (Sen, 2000). When we take a look at the lives of sexual minorities in the society, we can see that this is generally the case. They are typically excluded from typical family matters, connections, and decision-making processes inside their families; as a result, they are not involved in bigger society issues. This condition of Sexual minorities in the society has inspired the researcher's deep concern about the issue and motivated them to undertake the present research study. Despite the fact that the Indian constitution guarantees that "equality before the law regardless of their caste, religion, place of residence, gender, and sexuality," sexual minorities are treated inhumanely.

The many nomenclatures used to refer to people who are members of sexual minorities can lead to confusion and misunderstanding among the general public. The term "sexual minorities" refers to a group of people who do not belong to the majority culture. This group includes people who identify as lesbian, gay, bisexual, transgender, intersex, queer, female-to-male (FTM), male-to-female (MTF), and queer. It also includes culturally sanctioned labels like "queer" and "intersex.

Even though the people who fall into the categories of Hijra (Akwa and Nirvana), Kothi, Panti, Chakkas, Kinnar, Iravanis, Double Decker, Jogtas, Jogappa, Khusras, and Shiv-shaktis etc. have differences in their sexual orientation, sexual behavior, and occupation, among other things, the present study recognizes all of these groups collectively as members of a Sexual Minority. This chapter provides a brief introduction to two different concepts. The first concept is about the sexual minority community, including its history and origin, as well as studies and theories related to gender variant identity, the social and legal status of sexual minorities in India, the sexual minority population, and discrimination in the health care system, among other topics. The second concept is about how sexual minorities are treated unfairly. The second idea relates to social exclusion, which covers a wide range of topics including the meaning and definition of social exclusion, as well as its dimensions or indicators and how it is measured. The social marginalization of the sexual minority community, the justification for the study, and some concluding observations come to an end this chapter.

Understanding Sexual Minorities is the First Step.

The word "sexual minorities" is an umbrella term that embraces the several heterogeneous groups that are referred to as "the L.G.B.T population" together. These groups include lesbians, gays, bisexuals, and transgender people. Sexual minorities are groups of people whose sexual identities, orientations, or behaviors are distinct from those of the majority of the culture that surrounds them. Individuals who identify as Lesbian, Gay, Bisexual, or Transgender are typically included in the category of sexual minorities. (PUCL-K-2001) [Note: The term "sexual minority community" or "sexual minorities" refers to individuals who identify as lesbian, gay, bisexual, or transgendered/transsexual, in addition to other individuals who have different identities, such as kothis, pantis, hijras, double deckers, jogappas, etc., and who constitute a minority group within a total population that is dominated by heterosexuals (people who identify as cis gender). Who exactly are the LGBT? The term "Sexual Minorities" refers to the collective of identities that includes lesbians, gays, bisexuals, and transgender people A person is considered to be lesbian if they identify as a woman and have significant (to themselves) sexual or romantic interests towards another woman, or if they identify as a member of the lesbian community. This phrase can also be used to refer to women who identify as bisexual in India. (The CHLET 2012)

A person is said to be homosexual if they either self-identify as a member of the LGBT community or if they have significant (to themselves) sexual or romantic inclinations that are primarily directed toward individuals of the same gender or sex. a person who identifies with the LGBT community. It is possible to identify as a member of the homosexual community without also identifying as a gay individual, and vice versa. People who identify as men and are attracted to other people who identify as men are frequently referred to as "gay," despite the fact that the term "gay" is commonly used to refer to all homosexual individuals. males who identify as gay may not always engage in sexual activity just with other males; on occasion, they may also engage in sexual activity with women. (The CHLET 2012)

A person is said to be bisexual if they have romantic, emotional, and sexual attraction to both men and women. (The CHLET 2012) People who do not identify with or prefer not to comply to the gender roles that are ascribed to them by society based on their biological sex are referred to as transgender (TG). This is a broad term that encompasses all of these individuals. People are considered to be transgender if they break the gender norms of the society to which they belong and/or if they express or present a breaking and/or blurring of culturally prevalent or stereotypical gender roles. Transgender is often used as an umbrella term to refer to all people who defy rigid, binary gender constructions and who express or present a breaking and/or blurring of culturally prevalent gender roles. This includes a wide range of identities and experiences, including but not limited to the following: pre-operative, post-operative, and non-operative transsexual people; male and female cross dressers (sometimes referred to as transvestites, drag queens, or drag kings); intersex individuals; and men and women, regardless of their sexual orientation, whose appearance or characteristics are perceived to be gender atypical. (According to CHLET 2012, a person who transitions from being male to female is referred to as a transgender woman, and a person who transitions from being female to male is referred to as a transgender man.)

On the other hand, in Indian society, members of sexual minorities are generally acknowledged by names that are culturally sanctioned, such as Hijra. The term "hijra" comes from an Urdu-Hindustani word that derives from the Semitic Arabic root word "hjr," which has the sense of "leaving one's tribe." The term "hijra" was first used in the 7th century. Hijras are biologically males but have a feminine gender identity; they identify as female, wear women's clothing, and play roles that are traditionally associated with women. Hijras typically have their own distinct social and cultural identity, and they are also a part of a singular history that spans 4,000 years and represents an alternative society that has existed on the Indian mainland. The majority of hijras fall into one of two groups, and the name of their particular category reveals something about who they are as a being. The first type is known as Hijras (Akwa), and members of this group have not been castrated. Castration refers to the act of removing a man's testicles or another component of his sexual organs.

- person/animal) and as a result, they are permitted to engage in penetrative sex with both men and women. The second category of Nirvana Hijras consists of those who have been ritually castrated.

- The communities of Hijras are divided into seven primary clans that are collectively referred to as 'Gharanas.' These seven Gharanas are as follows:

- The Gharana of the Bhindi Bazar.

- The Delhi branch of the Gharana.

SEXUAL MINORITY 43

- Haidar Ibrahim, a member of the Gharana.

- The Gharana of Lucknow (Lucknow walla).

- Poona walla Gharana is the fifth.

- the sixth Gharana, the Lalan walla.

- The Bulack tribe of the Gharana.

The Sexual Minority community in the research area (Hubballi-Dharwad City) belongs to the "Poona walla" Gharana, and every "Gharana" is headed by a "Nayak," who is a key person and an elder Hijra. Under every Nayaka are many "Gurus," who are the teachers or masters, and every guru is having many "Chelas," which, in English, we call it as disciples. The majority of them do not live with their biological families either because their families choose to desert them owing to the fact that their gender identity is not accepted by society or because they themselves have chosen to become a part of the community. (2008) According to Anasuya Ray

The Gender Enigma or Paradox.

In biological organisms, the genetic and environmental factors play an essential role in the formation of sexual traits. Although there are two sexes in nature (namely, male and female), hermaphrodites, also known as bisexuals, can sometimes arise in the position of either one or both sexes. Only a few species do not have a predetermined sexual orientation, however this can shift in response to various cues. In light of this, there is a pressing need for the scientific community to acquire a comprehensive understanding of the intricacies involved in the process of determining sexuality throughout the diverse animal kingdom. In spite of this, genetics are responsible for sex determination in the vast majority of cases. Males and females of a species will typically have different alleles or a greater number of genes than are required to define definitive sexual morphology. In addition, the development of reproductive organs in human beings is largely dependent on the interactions between genes and the communication between cells. within the embryo itself, as well as with any other embryos that may be present in the uterus, as well as with the environment of the mother. 2014 according to Agoramoorthy

People who do not fit neatly into either the masculine or female category are referred to as transgender, third sex, or third gender in the anthropological community. These terms have been employed by some academics to define the sexual orientation, while others have suggested that this describes a male spirit inhabiting a female body. People of the third gender are referred to using a variety of regional and local names in different parts of the world, such as Hijras in South Asia, Berdache in North America, Xanith in the Arabian Peninsula, Female Husbands in West Africa, Sambia Boys in Papua New Guinea, Fa'afafine in Polynesia, Sworn Virgins in the Balkans, and

Katoey (lady boys) in Thailand. There was a time when the majority of countries in the western half of the world regarded the roles and behaviors that persons who identified as third gender followed as being unusual or rare. In spite of this, there has never been a consensus reached in the scientific literature regarding issues relating to gender. 2014 according to Agoramoorthy The preceding discussion (the Gender paradox/Enigma) is not sufficient to understand the facts behind the formation of gender role or characteristics of an individual; consequently, before looking into the history and origin of the Sexual Minority community, it is necessary to look into the various studies and theories related to Gender variant identity for the purpose of gaining a better understanding of the Sexual Minorities and their community.

Research dealing with gender identity in its many forms.

The distinctions between Sexual Minorities and Gender Minorities are not always clear to people, and they are frequently misunderstood. In general, those categories are included in the group of sexual minorities. Some examples of these groups are gays and lesbians, whose sexual orientation is towards their own biological sex. However, when it comes to gender minorities, these individuals are those who feel and express themselves in a manner that is contrary to their biological sex. Examples of these individuals include trans-woman

(MTF), trans-man (FTM), intersex, and others. Parents of children with various gender identities were more likely to attempt to transform their children throughout the 1970s and 1980s than they were to learn to accept their children in their natural state. Some of the academics and specialists in the field of mental health have come up with a theory on youngsters who have persistent and different gender preferences. This theory includes the guys who play at being female characteristics like Snow White and dress up like girls to express their desire to be a girl, among other behaviors. Were more prone to develop Gender Identity Disorder (GID) and look into transitioning into the opposite gender.

personal pronoun. According to the Diagnostic and Statistical Manual of Mental Disorders (DSM), the clinical term for the abnormal gender development is gender identity disorder (GID). (Academic Press, Compendium 2006) This is a relatively uncommon condition in which a person's gender identification (the psychological experience of oneself as to male or female) is the same as their phenotype (the external sex features of the body). This is regarded to be a rare disorder. Gender dysphoria refers to the personal discomfort that an individual has as a result of their gender identity. This condition, in its purest and most unrelenting form, is referred to as transsexualism. The persons who have experienced gender dysphoria have been raised in the gender role of boy or girl (boy or girl: the social category of gender), which is consistent with the external sex characteristics of their body; nonetheless, instances in which these individuals believe that they are psychologically different from their phenotypic are uncommon. They experience difficulty as a result of the social gender role as well as the exterior characteristics associated with their sexuality. In contrast, the majority of people grow up with very little or no distinction between their exterior sex characteristics, gender identity, their social roles as boy and girl, and their gender of raising. This is because the majority of people are raised by both biological mothers and biological fathers. (Haldeman, 2012) [Haldeman]

Research has been conducted in the topic of studying the gender-bending behaviors of individuals, and these studies have produced some interesting findings. In the modern academic world, studies that have been conducted on the stages of psychosocial development of children reveal that environmental influences play the most important role in the establishment of a child's gender identity. Transgender or gender variant people, on the other hand, violate the fundamental notion of these stereotypical binary gender roles, which contradicts the findings of these studies. There are parts of the world in which the existence of more than two distinct genders and gender roles, as well as the acceptance of those identities, is commonplace. The adjectives masculinity and femininity are used to describe gender the vast majority of the time; this is a societal explanation that differs across different cultures and over the course of history. We are able to identify the various civilizations that have a gender fluidity in their society. The categories of heterosexuality and homosexuality, as well as those of male and female, may not always provide a clear and unambiguous division of sex and gender. In South Asia, they are known as Hijras; in North America, they are known as Berdache; in the Arabian Peninsula, they are known as Xanith; and in Thailand, they are known as Katoey, which literally translates to "lady boys." These are all examples of various gender classifications that are distinct from the usual western split of persons into male and female. In addition, in some indigenous cultures in North America, the concept of gender is viewed more as a continuum than as a set of discrete classifications. Two-spirited people, who have characteristics and qualities that are traditionally associated with either gender, are held in particularly high esteem in these groups. It should come as no surprise that many cultures have adopted various

techniques to construct gender divergences, with varying degrees of acknowledgment of the gender's propensity to be complex and evolve over time. The morphological and endocrine explanations have both been included into biological theory over the course of its development. The consequences of congenital adrenal hyperplasia examination, which is an inherited condition of adrenal steroid genesis, have been used to study the relationship between the behavior of hormonal interactions in human beings. This condition is known as congenital adrenal hyperplasia.

Dorner proposed that gender identity disorder or ailment, as well as homosexual orientation in male individuals, is the result of a primarily female differentiated brain as well as a central nervous system Pseudo Hermaphroditism, which is caused by an absolute or relative androgen deficiency during the critical hypothalamic organizational phase in prenatal life. This phase is considered to be the most important time for the development of the hypothalamus. It was Doner in 1976. In their investigation of the causes of gender atypicality and sexual orientation, Zucker and Bradely presented a comprehensive overview of findings on neuro-endocrine and brain morphology. They have made an effort to address the difficult variables linked with the multifarious character of GID (Gender Identity Disorder) by recognising the interacting influence of constitutional predispositions and environmental effects. This is part of the effort they have made to address these variables. (2009) (Zucker, 1995)

In conventional explanations of biological phenomena, biologists have looked for anatomical and hormonal differences between male and female individuals in order to provide an explanation for the observed behavioral differences between the sexes. The fundamental assumptions that underlie this paradigm are that the structure of the brain is unchanging and permanent once it has been organized, that there are two types of brains—male and female—and that these two types of brains have structure that does not overlap in such a way that they can distinguish men and women from one another, and that there are two sorts of people. Chromosomes are a key factor in the gender identification of gender nonconforming people because of the crucial function that they play in the process. People who are born with only one or more than two sex chromosomes, such as 47XXX or 47 XXY (known as sex polysomies) or 45X or 45Y (known as sex monosomies), are referred to as having gender variant chromosomes. This topic is the subject of a significant amount of controversy. There have been isolated instances of males being born with 46XX due to the translocation of a very little portion of the sex-determining region off of the Y chromosomes. Likewise, in the circumstances of the females who were born with 46XY chromosomes, this is the situation. However, the individuals listed above are not the only ones who have those particular sorts of chromosomal pairing; there is also a wide variety of hormones involved.

differences in chromosome complementarity, internal and exterior sex traits, and the overall balance are what determine sex. Sandra Bem presented the gender schema theory in 1981. It is an analytical theory that explains how an individual is assigned a gender by the society in which they live, as well as how sex-linked characteristics are preserved and transmitted to other cultures. According to this idea, gender-related information is primarily disseminated across society by means of informational schemes or networks, which permits certain information to be more easily understood than other information. Sandra Bem goes on to explain that individuals will differ in the degree to which they hold such gender systems and adhere to them. Sandra Bem also discussed the various categories into which a person's sexual orientation can be classified, and these distinctions are reflected in the degree to which individuals are capable of being sex-typed. The information processing and combination done by sex-typed people is determined by their birth sex; on the other hand, cross-sex-typed people's information processing and combination is determined by the opposite of their birth sex. Androgynous people take characteristics and information from both genders and blend them in their own unique way. But this begs the question: are chromosomes the only factor that determines a person's gender, or does a person's upbringing also play a crucial influence in shaping their gender identity? (Bem, 1981)

The psychoanalytic theory proposed by Sigmund Freud states that children go through a number of different phases of psychosocial development. Freud had portrayed in a very vivid manner the behavior and degree of sexual desire in children as they went through the stages of their development. It was common practice to use the terms "Oedipus Complex" and "Electra Complex" when attempting to characterize the mental state of a child who was in the phallic stage of psychosocial development. The genitals are the primary focus of libido during the phallic stage of development. Children of this age also begin to become aware of the differences between girls and boys and the roles that each plays in society. Freud published his work in

1957. A well-known Psychologist by the name of Karen Horney disagreed with the psychoanalysis idea, arguing that it was both wrong and offensive to women. As an alternative, Karen Horney proposed that men experience emotions of inferiority due to the fact that men are unable to give birth to offspring. Horney referred to this phenomenon as "womb envy." 2015 according to Cherry.

The psychosexual behavior of youngsters who find themselves to be the polar opposite of their own sex is not highlighted by the theory, which is a limitation of the theory. The culture of the theory is so heavily influenced by western culture that it cannot be applied to eastern cultures. According to the social learning theory developed by Albert Bandura, children acquire appropriate social behavior through imitation of the role models that are already established in society. It relies heavily on rewarding desirable behavior and penalizing undesirable behavior. The same learning principles that influence the learning of other types of behaviors are also responsible for the development of sexually oriented behaviors. In point of fact, sex-typed behaviors are defined as "behaviors that generally bring out different rewards for one sex than for the other" (Behaviors that generally bring out different rewards for one sex than for the other). Because boys and girls experience various outcomes, their sex-typical behaviors develop diverse meanings and manifest themselves at varying rates depending on the gender. As a result, the disparities in behavior that are observed between males and girls are fully attributable to the distinct conditioning experiences that they have had. A youngster will initially learn how to discriminate, just like they will with other sorts of learning. The individual eventually acquires the capacity to differentiate between gender-typical patterns of behavior. According to Michel (1966), whether a person identifies as male or female relies on the physical, social, and psychological similarities and differences that exist between the sexes.

A youngster will develop a sense of their own gender identity in part as a result of making comparisons between their own behavioral repertoire and the repertoires of the people in their immediate environment. 2006 according to Factor Cognitive Development Theory: A cognitive developmental account of gender development differs from both psychoanalytic accounts and social learning accounts in its premise that self-categorization as a boy or a girl, also known as gender identity, is the basis upon which sex-roles are learnt. This is where the cognitive developmental account of gender development departs from both psychoanalytic accounts and social learning accounts. The realization that one is a member of one of two dichotomous sexes is the aspect of gender development that takes place chronologically earliest and is the most fundamental. 2006 according to Factor

The proponents of queer theory are of the belief that one's gender identity is not a fixed or rigid identity, but rather, one's gender identity is something that can continue to develop and change over the course of time. Queer theory developed as a response to the anticipated constraints of the way in which identifications tend to get amalgamated or stable (for example, homosexual or straight). Additionally, theorists interpreted queerness in an attempt to oppose this tendency. Rather than attempting to define a particular identity in this manner, the theory aimed to uphold a critique. The term "queer" has a straightforward meaning, and it is frequently utilized to convey the idea of an identity that is not rigidly constructed but is, rather, malleable and subject to change. (2014) According to Boundless. Many psychologists claim that society and culture have a substantial part in determining the gender of the kid; nevertheless, people of atypical gender or gender variant break this notion of the impact of social and cultural influence on them and demonstrate that gender is not determined solely by the environment in which the child is raised.

Put into doubt the results of the most important studies on how society and culture are related to gender identification. Both twins were born in Canada; both were boys, and during a medical procedure one of the boys, Bruce, had been engaged in an accident, and the penis had been burned in the procedure. The author discusses the extremely well-known case of John and Joan, in which the twins' names were Bruce and Brian Reimer, and they were born in Canada. After consulting with a therapist, Bruce's parents made the decision to bring him up under the guise of a female called Brenda. But she was not like other girls in terms of her temperament; for example, she was assertive and dominant, and as time went on, she had fewer friends as she reached her teenage years. She was referred to as a cavewoman in the past. Later on, when she discovered her sex at the time of her birth, she made the decision to change both her sex and her gender identity. She even married a woman after making the transition. This instance demonstrates the significance of society in the process of deciding an individual's gender. (Reporter, 2010) [Reference] An investigation investigating the effects of feminizing intersex surgery on the sexual function of adults who were born with ambiguous genitalia was carried out in 2003 by Minto and her colleagues, amongst other researchers. There is no evidence that feminizing genital surgery leads to improved psycho-social outcomes; however, feminizing genital surgery cannot guarantee that adult gender identity will develop as a female; and that adult sexual function might be altered by removal of clitoral or phallic tissue. These are the findings of this study, which found that a number of moral issues in regards to the surgery include the following: there is no proof that feminizing genital surgery leads to the improved psycho-social outcomes.

In her book titled "Gender Trouble," author Judith Butler makes the argument that the feminist movement made a mistake when it attempted to establish that women were a community that shared common interests and characteristics. The author also stated that they performed "an unwitting regulation and reification of gender relations," which reinforced a binary view of gender relations in which people are primarily separated into two major groups, namely men and women. Therefore, feminism had the opposite effect of what it intended, which was to restrict people's ability to establish and select their own unique identities rather than opening up choices in this regard. In other words, the author suggested that gender should not be considered a constant feature in an individual but rather as a flexible variable that shifts and changes in different settings and at different durations, rather than treating gender as if it were a stable attribute. One of the most important ideas in queer theory is that identification is something that can be free-floating and is not tied to an essence but is instead something that can be performed. When viewed in this light, our identities, regardless of whether they are gendered or not, do not convey any genuine aspect of our inner selves; rather, they are the dramatic effect (rather than the cause) of our performances. (2002) Butler's findings.

Reflections on sex, gender, sexuality, psychoanalysis, and medical care of intersex people were the primary topics covered in Judith Butler's book "Undoing Gender," which was written for a wider audience and targeted specifically at common readers. The author examines and improves our understanding of the concept of performativity while concentrating on the challenge of removing normatively limiting conceptions of sexual and gendered life. The author explained how gender is performed without one being conscious of it; yet, just because this occurs without one's awareness does not indicate that this performativity is automatic or mechanical. The author goes on to claim that people have desires that do not arise from their personality but rather from the societal standards that they were raised with. The author also questions our conception of what it means to be human and what it means to be less than human, as well as how conceptions that are imposed by culture might prevent a person from living a viable life. The most common worry is whether or not a person will be accepted if their desires deviate from what is considered normal. According to the author, a person could sense the need to be identified in order to continue living, but at the same time, the requirements that must be met to be recognized render existence unlivable. The author suggests doing an investigation into such circumstances in order to provide individuals who defy them with additional opportunities for life. (2009) (Butler, 2004)

Within the context of her study of intersex, author Judith Butler refers to the example of David Reimer, a person whose genitalia were surgically altered from male to female following an unsuccessful circumcision when the individual was eight months old. David Reimer was born male but was given the female gender by physicians when he was young. Later in life, he realized his true gender, married, and became the stepfather to his wife's three children. After some time, Reimer took his own life. However, it is possible to draw a number of different conclusions regarding the gender development of a person based on the ongoing discussion that has been taking place above regarding the studies and theories that are related to the gender variant identities. These conclusions can be drawn as a result of the ongoing discussion on the studies and theories that are related to the gender variant identities. Coming to a consensus on a single body of research or idea is an extremely challenging process. As a result, all of the significant studies and theories associated with gender variant identities have been covered up to this point. In the next section, we will talk about the history of the sexual minority group in India.

History of Sexual Minorities in India.

Without considering the Hindu concept of a 'Third sex,' also known as Tritiya prakriti or Third nature, any debate made on Sexual Minorities or the number of Third Gender individuals would not be considered to be full. The 'Kama Sutra,' which was written in the fourth century and is considered a sacred scripture on sexuality, emphasizes satisfaction as the primary goal of sexual encounters. It is a classification. It further subclassifies men who wish another man as a 'Third nature' into feminine and masculine types, and it also explains their lives and jobs (for example, masseurs, flower vendors, and hairdressers).

In this section, we will talk about the history of sexual minorities and the population of people who identify as third gender in ancient, medieval, and modern Indian civilization. Hinduism, also known as the Hindu religion, is considered to be the oldest of all the prominent religions in the world; its origins can be traced all the way back to 5000 BC. Today, more than 900 million people throughout the world practice Hinduism. However, the most important aspect of Hinduism is the trinity of gods, which is represented by Lord Brahma (the creator), Lord Vishnu (the protector), and Lord Shiva (the destroyer). There are roughly 33 crore deities that make up the complete pantheon of Hindus (all the gods of Hindus, collectively). Lord Vishnu is famous for his multiple incarnations, also known as avatars. Some of these avatars take the appearance of animals, such as the fish (Matayavatar) and the boar (Varahavatara), while others take the form of people, such as Lord Rama in the Ramayana and Lord Kishna in the Mahabharata.

According to Hindu mythology, a long time ago there was a hero named Iravan (also known as Aravan), who was one of these minor yet crucial characters of the Mahabharata, who was intended to marry Mohini through self-sacrifice before his death, this was as the boon given by the goddess Kali, to accomplish the boon, Lord Krishna (one of the avatars of Vishnu, Lord Krishna was the charioteer of King Arjuna in After that, Mohini transformed back into Lord Krishna. This transition ceremony is something that the sexual minority (Hijra) population in India looks forward to celebrating every year. The same thing happened to Arjuna, and she transitioned into a transgender person as well. When Arjuna turned down Urvashi's proposal of marriage when he was exiled, she became enraged and cursed him to transition into the other gender out of spite. Historians are of the belief that this event led to Arjuna's transformation into a transgender person. The disheartened Arjuna got perplexed about the impending curse of Urvashi. Lord Vishnu came and convinced Arjuna that a transgender makeover would produce a helpful disguise as Arjuna had to complete his exile away from his country. Arjuna then thanked Lord Vishnu and took a bow before leaving. he took on the name Brihannala, traveled to a distant nation for a year, and at the end of that time he was reborn as a man. Similarly, one of Lord Shiva's appearances includes Ardhanari, which is half man and half woman divided in the middle, and statues of this mark can still be seen in many of the Hindu temples. Additionally, a popular deity worshiped in south India called Lord Ayyappa was the result of a homosexual union between two male gods, Lord Shiva and Lord Vishnu. Lord Ayyappa is believed to have been created by Lord Shiva and Lord Vishnu.

The history of hijras dates back to the beginning of humankind. The presence of the Hijras was made known in the Hindu scriptures known as the 'Vedas' and the 'Granthas'. It is believed that the inhabitants of the Ayodhya Kingdom gathered to bid farewell to Lord Ram, Sita, and Laxman before they were sent into exile for fourteen years by Lord Ram's father, King Dashratha, in accordance with the demand made by King Dashratha's third wife, Kaikai. The folks followed them as they made their way toward the 'Vanavasa' as they were departing. Then Lord Ram commanded his subjects to come back, calling them as men and women (He 'Nar Nari Tum JaSakte-Ho), but in addition to the men and women, the Hijras who were living in that era and were referred to as 'Sikhandi' were also there. They remained there for fourteen years until Lord Ram returned, despite the fact that Lord Ram had ordered them to return, since their allegiance to Lord Ram was so strong that he did not consider them to be either men or women and so did not order them to home. The Hijras were the ones who carried out the practice of "Tapasya" in its truest form. They went fourteen years without eating or drinking anything at all. It was only after this episode that Lord Ram bestowed upon them the "Vardana," which ensured that whenever there was a joyous occasion, such as a wedding or the birth of a child, people would always remember to send them an invitation. Since that time, their significance in Indian culture has become increasingly apparent. It is reported in the 'Mahabharata' that Arjuna was unable to overcome Bhishmapitamaha, the leader of the Kauravas, during the battle of 'Kurukshetra' between the Pandavas and the Kauravas. Then, Bhishmapitamaha asserted that the only way to defeat him was to bring before him a "Sikhandi," a man who was not entirely male and so would never be the target of his sword. Then Arjun did take refuge behind a Sikhandi (it is stated in the Mahabharata that the Hijras that existed during that period were called as Sikhandis), on whom Bhishmapitamaha did not raise his sword. It is stated that this was the one and only factor that contributed to the Pandavas' victory in the Mahabharata conflict. (Written by Veena N.A. Goswami)

The aforementioned accounts of transgenders existing and being involved in prominent deities are well approved of and accepted by the millions of Hindus who practice the religion. As a result, it is abundantly clear that the Hindu faith has surpassed other religions across the globe in terms of the concerns pertaining to social acceptance of homosexuality and transgenderism as valid identities in our culture. The concept of a god who is either female or male or who is gender neutral is one that continues to receive approval and acceptance among Hindus. There was no stigma attached to having a Hijra in ancient India. In today's world, however, the situation is exactly the opposite; people have cast these individuals out of society not due to the fact that they are social outcasts, but rather due to the abnormalities that they exhibit in their sexual organs. In addition, throughout the Mughal Empire (1504–1719), transgender people have played an important role as royal guards in the courtyards of Mughal palaces. This practice dates back to the Middle Ages. However, this condition of transgender people did not begin to deteriorate until the rule of British rule in India (1757–1947). In India, the colonial administrators initiated the Section 377 of the IPC (Indian Penal Code) in 1860, which proclaimed homosexuality to be a criminal activity and similarly listed transgender people as criminal elements in society. During this time, the condition of transgender people did not improve. This harmful law remained on the books for close to 149 years, right up until it was finally overturned in 2009, which was extremely recently. 2014 according to Agoramoorthy

In the modern era, people who belong to sexual minorities or who transition between genders can be found all over India. They are known by a variety of names in the area, such as Chakkas, Hijras, Kothis, Kinnars, Iravanis, Jogtas, Jogappas, Shiv-shaktis, and Khusras. They are also known for their exuberance and the colorful female garb that they wear when they are seen in public. This one-of-a-kind cultural minority has repeatedly been disregarded and disregarded as irrelevant by the normal traditionalist culture. Nirvana, also known as the sex reassignment surgery, is performed on a significant number of biological males (Hijras) in the form of a ritualized castration. They are comparable to biological hermaphrodites in that they are born with genitalia that are ambiguously male-like. The precise number of people who identify as members of sexual minorities or who identify as transgender is unknown, but census data collecting agencies have historically neglected the existence of sexual minority populations in their work. In spite of this, a variety of non-governmental social work organizations in India have attempted to estimate the country's transgender population, which may reach as high as six million people. In October 2013, the Supreme Court of India made the statement that members of the sexual minority or the transgender population have been treated as untouchables by society due to their limited access to health care, education, and employment opportunities. During a hearing of a PIL (Public Interest Litigation) brought by the National Legal Services Authority, the judges of India's Supreme Court reprimanded the government for the presence of such discrimination against them. The PIL was filed in response to a lawsuit in the public interest. This judicial organization advocates for the rights of those who identify as belonging to sexual minority groups. That sexual minorities cannot be discriminated against on the basis of their sex, and that they do, in fact, fall under the social and educational backward classification specified in Article 15 (4) of the Indian Constitution is a question that has been raised by social activists

Its founding document. The highest court in India has issued an order to the country's federal government, instructing them to place members of the transgender population under the category of "other backward classes" (OBCs), which indicates a more socially and economically disadvantaged standing in Indian society. The court has ordered all of India's states to build public restrooms that are gender-specifically designated for transgender people. Additionally, the Supreme Court issued an order directing the government to establish welfare groups in order to improve the individuals' health and meet their medical requirements. After rethinking the Supreme Court's decision, the highest level of government went back to the court to seek further clarification. In its request, it emphasized that it would be impractical to classify sexual minorities alongside OBCs, given that some of them may already have been included in OBCs. On the other hand, the central government admitted that they could be counted as OBCs if the National Commission for Backward Classes (NCBC) deems it to be an essential measure. In addition, the central government has asked the Supreme Court for clarity on the meaning of the term "transgender," which might refer to the entire lesbian, gay, bisexual, and transgender population. However, according to the legal experts, the fact that the court's judgment specifically included the transgender population means that the court's verdict does not encompass lesbians, gays, or bisexuals. For close to two centuries, transgender people have been marginalized in terms of their ability to participate in social and cultural life. Even at the present day, they have limited access to public facilities, educational opportunities, and medical care. To make matters even worse, they are treated as nonentity legally, which is in fact the clear violation of the Indian Constitution. This is a clear breach of the Indian Constitution. The residents of the nation are granted the right to vote as well as the opportunity to run for office by virtue of the constitution of the country. However, before to the year 1993, voters could only choose between male and female candidates on their election ballots.

It wasn't until the year 1994 that authorities were finally given the opportunity to participate in the voting process for the very first time in elections. This was made possible since the electoral commission of India created a third gender category known as E (eunuch) to acknowledge authorities as citizens of the nation. Some of them are running for the position of member of parliament in the general elections that will take place in the year 2014 in their respective regions. However, until the society as a whole makes some concerted efforts, transgender people in India might not be able to exercise their democratic rights in areas such as marriage, the adoption and upbringing of children, and the utilization of economic support systems such as free and subsidized medical treatments, health care, and surgeries. It is thought that almost 25 percent of transgender individuals have been issued national identification cards (Aadhaar) by UDAI (Unique Identification Authority of India), although there is evidence to suggest that this number is far lower. It is still difficult for transgender people to obtain ration cards, national income tax permanent account numbers (PAN), and driving licenses, all of which are required to receive government assistance. In recent years, advocates for human rights have been campaigning for transgender people to be granted legal recognition.

Two

Sexology

The term "sexology" does not typically relate to the non-scientific study of sexuality, such as social critique, but rather to the scientific study of human sexuality, which includes human sexual interests, behaviors, and functions. [1] Sexology is the scientific study of human sexuality, which includes human sexual interests, behaviors, and functions. Tools from a variety of academic disciplines, including anthropology, biology, medicine, psychology, epidemiology, sociology, and criminology, are utilized by sexologists. [4][5] Some of the topics that are investigated by sexologists are sexual development (puberty), sexual orientation, gender identity, sexual relationships, sexual activities, paraphilias, and atypical sexual interests. In addition to this, it encompasses the study of sexuality at all stages of a person's life, from childhood through adulthood, including puberty, adolescent sexuality, and sexuality in older adults. In addition, sexology encompasses sexuality among those who have mental or physical impairments. Mainstays also include the investigation of sexual dysfunctions and disorders, such as erectile dysfunction and anorgasmia, via the lens of sexology.

Early on

Since ancient times, people have written guides on how to enjoy sexual encounters. Some of these guides include Ovid's Ars Amatoria, the Kama Sutra of Vatsyayana, the Ananga Ranga, and The Perfumed Garden for the Recreation of the Soul. Prostitution in the City of Paris, which was written by Alexander Jean Baptiste Parent-Duchatelet in the early 1830s and published in 1837, a year after he died, is considered to be the first work of modern sex research. [2] In England, James Graham was an early sexologist who lectured on subjects such as the process of sex and conception. [The scientific study of sexual behavior in human beings began in the 19th century with Heinrich Kaan. Michel Foucault describes Kaan's book Psychopathia Sexualis (1844) as marking "the date of birth, or in any case the date of the emergence of sexuality and sexual aberrations in the psychiatric field." [7] Elizabeth Osgood Goodrich Willard coined the term "sexology" for the first time in the United States in 1867. Roughly simultaneously

- From the Victorian era right up until World War II

- Havelock Ellis was a forerunner in the drive toward sexual liberation in the late 19th century. He is known as "the father of the suffragettes."

The drive toward sexual emancipation started towards the end of the nineteenth century in England and Germany, in spite of the prevalent social attitude of sexual repression that existed during the Victorian era. The book "Psychopathia Sexualis" was written by Richard Freiherr von Krafft-Ebing and published in 1886. This body of studies is credited with laying the groundwork for sexology as a field within the scientific community.

Havelock Ellis, a physician and sexologist, is considered to be the founding father of sexology in England. He was a pioneer in the field by challenging the sexual taboos of his time period, particularly those pertaining to homosexuality and masturbation, and he altered how people thought about sex throughout his era. The Sexual Inversion, which he published in 1897, is considered to be his primary work. It details the sexual relationships of homosexual males, including those between men and youngsters. Ellis is credited with having written the first objective study of homosexuality (Karl-Maria Kertbeny was the one who came up with the word "homosexuality"). Ellis did not view homosexuality as an illness, as something immoral, or as a criminal. The book makes the assumption that age taboos and gender taboos around same-sex love have been overcome. Seven out of his total of twenty-one case studies focus on connections spanning many generations. He also established other significant psychological concepts, such as autoeroticism and narcissism, both of which were later explored further by Sigmund Freud. [10] Among his other contributions to the field of psychology, he is most known for his theory of the unconscious. Together with the German Magnus Hirschfeld, Ellis was one of the pioneers of the transgender phenomenon. He established it as a new category that was separate and distinct from homosexuality. [11] Ellis, who was aware of Hirschfeld's studies of transvestism but disagreed with his terminology, proposed the term sexo-aesthetic inversion to characterize the phenomenon in 1913. He was aware of Hirschfeld's investigations of transvestism.

Journal of Sexology, also known as Zeitschrift for Sexualwissenschaft, was the first academic journal to be published in the discipline. It began publishing in 1908 and continued publishing once a month for an entire year. These issues featured writing by Freud, Alfred Adler, and Wilhelm Stekel[3]. In 1913, the first academic society dedicated to the study of sexology was established; it was called the Society for Sexology. Freud was the first person to establish a theory of sexuality. Oral, anal, phallic, latency, and genital are the phases that make up this progression of development. Based on his observations of his clients throughout the latter part of the 19th century and the early part of the 20th century, he determined that these stages extend from childhood through puberty and beyond. Freud's students Wilhelm Reich and Otto Gross were opposed to his ideas because they placed an emphasis on the part that sexuality played in the revolutionary battle for the emancipation of mankind. Freud's theories were rejected for this reason. Books written by Hirschfeld were considered "un-German" by Nazis in Berlin, therefore they were destroyed.

Under the impact of the sexually progressive Napoleonic code, pre-Nazi Germany organized and fought against the anti-sexual cultural forces of Victorian England. As a result of the momentum generated by such groups, sex research was coordinated across traditional academic fields in Germany, propelling the country to the forefront of the sexology field. Magnus Hirschfeld, a physician, was a vocal supporter of sexual minorities and the founder of the Scientific Humanitarian Committee, which was the first organization to campaign for the rights of homosexuals and transsexual people. [16] In the same year, 1919, Hirschfeld was also responsible for establishing the first Institut fur Sexualwissenschaft (Institute for Sexology) in Berlin. Over 20,000 books, 35,000 photos, and a substantial collection of art in addition to other things might be found within its library. People from all over Europe traveled to the institute in order to improve their awareness of their sexuality and receive treatment for sexual issues and dysfunctions they were experiencing.

Hirschfeld is credited with identifying a group of people that are today referred to as transsexual or transgender as separate from the categories of homosexuality; he referred to these people as transvestiten (transvestites). Germany's dominance in sexual behavior research led to Hirschfeld's development of a system that identified numerous actual or hypothetical types of sexual intermediary between heterosexual male and female to represent the potential diversity of human sexuality. Ernst Burchard and Benedict Friedlaender were two more sexologists who were involved in the early stages of the homosexual rights movement. Ernst Grafenberg, whose name is given to the G-spot on the map, was the researcher who first published the research that led to the development of the intrauterine device (IUD).

After the end of WWII

Following the conclusion of World War II, both the United States and Europe witnessed a revival in the field of sexology. Large-scale investigations of sexual behavior, sexual function, and sexual dysfunction gave rise to the development of sex therapy. [3] Post-World War II sexology in the United States was affected by the flood of European refugees escaping the Nazi government as well as the popularity of the Kinsey studies. Alfred Kinsey established the Institute for Sex Research at Indiana University in Bloomington in 1947. Prior to that time, the majority of American sexology consisted of organizations attempting to put an end to prostitution and to educate young people about sexually transmitted illnesses. [2] In 1947, Alfred Kinsey established the Institute for Sex Research. The Kinsey Institute for Research in Sex, Gender, and Reproduction is the current name for this organization. In the book that he published in 1948, he stated that more was known scientifically about the sexual behavior of farm animals than was known about people.In the 1950s, sexologist and psychologist John Money created theories on sexual identity as well as gender identity. Even though the David Reimer case was essential to the establishment of treatment regimens for intersex newborns and children, his work, particularly on that instance, has subsequently been seen as controversial. [20][21] [vague]

In the 1950s, a man named Kurt Freund worked in Czechoslovakia to develop the penile plethysmograph. The instrument was developed to give an objective measurement of sexual arousal in males and is currently used in the assessment of pedophilia and hebephilia. Its purpose was to provide an objective measurement of sexual arousal in males. Since then, this instrument has been utilized with sexual offenders. Masters and Johnson each published their book titled Human Sexual Response in 1966 and 1970, respectively. Johnson's book was titled Human Sexual Inadequacy. These books were successful in the marketplace, and in 1978, the authors were instrumental in establishing what would later be called the Masters and Johnson Institute.

- During this time period, Vern Bullough was active in the field of sexology research in addition to his role as a historian of sexology.

- The appearance of HIV/AIDS in the 1980s prompted a significant change in sexological research efforts toward the goal of comprehending and halting the progression of the disease.

century of the 21st

Studies including behavioral genetics[27], neuroimaging[28], and large-scale Internet-based surveys[29] are now able to be conducted as a result of technological advancements since they are able to address sexological questions. In some jurisdictions, the field of sexology is a professionally regulated occupation. Sexologists in the Canadian province of Quebec are required to be members of the Ordre professionnel des sexologues du Québec. Sexology is the scientific study of human sexuality, which includes human sexual interests, behaviors, and functions. The term "sexology" does not generally refer to the non-scientific study of sexuality, such as social criticism. It is one of the professions that are eligible to receive psychotherapy permits from the Ordre des psychologues du Québec. Tools from a variety of academic disciplines, including anthropology, biology, medicine, psychology, epidemiology, sociology, and criminology, are utilized by sexologists. [4][5] Some of the topics that are investigated by sexologists are sexual development (puberty), sexual orientation, gender identity, sexual relationships, sexual activities, paraphilias, and atypical sexual interests. In addition to this, it encompasses the study of sexuality at all stages of a person's life, from childhood through adulthood, including puberty, adolescent sexuality, and sexuality in older adults. In addition, sexology encompasses sexuality among those who have mental or physical impairments. Mainstays also include the investigation of sexual dysfunctions and disorders, such as erectile dysfunction and anorgasmia, via the lens of sexology

Since ancient times, people have written guides on how to enjoy sexual encounters. Some of these guides include Ovid's Ars Amatoria, the Kama Sutra of Vatsyayana, the Ananga Ranga, and The Perfumed Garden for the Recreation of the Soul. Prostitution in the City of Paris, which was written by Alexander Jean Baptiste Parent-Duchatelet in the early 1830s and published in 1837, a year after he died, is considered to be the first work of modern sex research. [2] In England, James Graham was an early sexologist who lectured on subjects such as the process of sex and conception. [6] The scientific study of sexual behavior in human beings began in the 19th century with Heinrich Kaan. Michel Foucault describes Kaan's book Psychopathia Sexualis (1844) as marking "the date of birth, or in any case the date of the emergence of sexuality and sexual aberrations in the psychiatric field." [7] Elizabeth Osgood Goodrich Willard coined the term "sexology" for the first time in the United States in 1867. Roughly simultaneously

- From the Victorian era right up until World War II

- Havelock Ellis was a forerunner in the drive toward sexual liberation in the late 19th century. He is known as "the father of the suffragettes."

The drive toward sexual emancipation started towards the end of the nineteenth century in England and Germany, in spite of the prevalent social attitude of sexual repression that existed during the Victorian era. The book "Psychopathia Sexualis" was written by Richard Freiherr von Krafft-Ebing and published in 1886. This body of studies is credited with laying the groundwork for sexology as a field within the scientific community Havelock Ellis, a physician and sexologist, is considered to be the founding father of sexology in England. He was a pioneer in the field by challenging the sexual taboos of his time period, particularly those pertaining to homosexuality and masturbation, and he altered how people thought about sex throughout his era. The Sexual Inversion, which he published in 1897, is considered to be his primary work. It details the sexual relationships of homosexual males, including those between men and youngsters. Ellis is credited with having written the first objective study of homosexuality (Karl-Maria Kertbeny was the one who came up with the word "homosexuality"). Ellis did not view homosexuality as an illness, as something immoral, or as a criminal. The book makes the assumption that age taboos and gender taboos around same-sex love have been overcome. Seven out of his total of twenty-one case studies focus on connections spanning many generations. He also established other significant psychological concepts, such as auto-eroticism and narcissism, both of which were later explored further by Sigmund Freud. [10] Among his other contributions to the field of psychology, he is most known for his theory of the unconscious. Together with the German Magnus Hirschfeld, Ellis was one of the pioneers of the transgender phenomenon. He established it as a new category that was separate and distinct from homosexuality. [11] Ellis, who was aware of Hirschfeld's studies of transvestism but disagreed with his terminology, proposed the term sexo-aesthetic inversion to characterize the phenomenon in 1913. [12][13] He was aware of Hirschfeld's investigations of transvestism. Journal of Sexology, also known as Zeitschrift for Sexualwissenschaft, was the first academic journal to be published in the discipline. It began publishing in 1908 and continued publishing once a month for an entire year. These issues featured writing by Freud, Alfred Adler, and Wilhelm Stekel[3]. In 1913, the first academic society dedicated to the study of sexology was established; it was called the Society for Sexology[14].Freud was the first person to establish a theory of sexuality. Oral, anal, phallic, latency, and genital are the phases that make up this progression of development. Based on his observations of his clients throughout the latter part of the 19th century and the early part of the 20th century, he determined that these stages extend from childhood through puberty and beyond. Freud's students Wilhelm Reich and Otto Gross were opposed to his ideas because they placed an emphasis on the part that sexuality played in the revolutionary battle for the emancipation of mankind. Freud's theories were rejected for this reason.

Under the impact of the sexually progressive Napoleonic code, pre-Nazi Germany organized and fought against the anti-sexual cultural forces of Victorian England. As a result of the momentum generated by such groups, sex research was coordinated across traditional academic fields in Germany, propelling the country to the forefront of the sexology field. Magnus Hirschfeld, a physician, was a vocal supporter of sexual minorities and the founder of the Scientific Humanitarian Committee, which was the first organization to campaign for the rights of homosexuals and transsexual people. [In the same year, 1919, Hirschfeld was also responsible for establishing the first Institut fur Sexualwissenschaft (Institute for Sexology) in Berlin. Over 20,000 books, 35,000 photos, and a substantial collection of art in addition to other things might be found within its library. People from all over Europe traveled to the institute in order to improve their awareness of their sexuality and receive treatment for sexual issues and dysfunctions they were experiencing. Hirschfeld is credited with identifying a group of people that are today referred to as transsexual or transgender as separate from the categories of homosexuality; he referred to these people as transvestiten (transvestites). Germany's dominance in sexual behavior research led to Hirschfeld's development of a system that identified numerous actual or hypothetical types of sexual intermediary between heterosexual male and female to represent the potential diversity of human sexuality. Ernst Burchard and Benedict Fried laender were two more sexologists who were involved in the early stages of the homosexual rights movement. Ernst Grafenberg, whose name is given to the G-spot on the map, was the researcher who first published the research that led to the development of the intrauterine device (IUD).

History of human sexuality

The research into the evolution of sexual behavior in humans.

Leonardo da Vinci's "Coition of a Hemisected Man and Woman" (about 1492) is an interpretation of what occurs inside the body during vaginal intercourse. It was completed around the year 1492 .Johann Bachofen was a Swiss lawyer whose work had a significant effect on the development of the study of the history of sexuality. Bachofen's thoughts on the topic, which were almost exclusively derived from an in-depth examination of ancient mythology, were attacked by a number of authors, the most notable of which being Lewis Henry Morgan and Friedrich Engels. Both of these authors were influenced by Bachofen. Bachofen claims in his book Mother Right: An Investigation of the Religious and Juridical Character of Matriarchy in the Ancient World that human sexuality was disorderly and promiscuous in the beginning of human history. Bachofen's book was published in 1861.

This matriarchal "aphroditic" stage gave way to a matriarchal "demeteric" stage as a result of the mother being the only reliable way of establishing descendants. The "aphroditic" stage was superseded by the "demeteric" stage. Only once humans switched to a system of monogamy that was imposed by men was it able to determine who the biological father of a child was. This was the beginning of patriarchy, the final "apolloan" stage of human evolution. Even though Bachofen's ideas are not supported by any empirical data, they are significant due to the influence they had on subsequent generations of intellectuals, particularly in the discipline of cultural anthropology.

The study of evolution, and more specifically the branch of biology known as human behavioral ecology, is the foundation for today's interpretations of where human sexuality came from. The study of evolutionary biology has demonstrated that the human genome, as well as the genotypes of all other animals, is the product of those ancestors who reproduced more frequently than other ancestors did. Because natural selection does not have the ability to "see" into the future, the resulting adaptations in sexual behavior are not a "attempt" on the part of the individual to maximize reproduction in a particular circumstance. On the other hand, it is more likely that the current behavior is the outcome of selection factors that took place during the Pleistocene. Clay plaque depicting sexual activity between a female and a male. 2000 B.C.E., in Mesopotamia For instance, a man who attempts to have sex with multiple women while avoiding the involvement of his parents is not acting in this manner because he wants to "increase his fitness." Rather, he is acting in this manner because the psychological framework that emerged and flourished during the Pleistocene era has persisted to this day[2].On a bed, sexual activity between a guy and a female. Model made of clay. Ancient Babylonian. The British Museum in London, circa the year 1800 BCE A vessel with paintings by Recuay. Clay used in terracotta. Peru. The Museum of the United States in Madrid. between 400 BCE and 300 CE.

The sources

Since the beginning of history, different criteria of decency have been applied to different forms of sexual speaking, and by implication, to sexual writing. Throughout the vast majority of historical time, writing was not utilized by more than a relatively small percentage of any society's total population. Because of this, there is a paucity of direct and reliable data on which to build a history due to the widespread practice of self-censorship and the proliferation of euphemism terms. The following are some examples of primary sources that can be gathered from a wide range of historical eras and cultural settings:

- Legislative history suggesting either promotion or restriction of the activity

- Texts from various religions and schools of thought that advocate for, oppose, or discuss the subject at hand

- Diaries and other forms of personal contact, as well as other literary sources, may have remained unpublished throughout the writers' lifetimes.

- The majority of medical encyclopedias classify various types as pathological conditions.

- Changes in language, notably in slang. linguistic advances.

- More recently, research on sexuality has focused on

- Sexuality in a variety of world cultures

- First Nations Peoples

George Caitlin (1796-1872) drew this depiction of a celebration ceremonial dance for a two spirit person while he was living among the Sac and Fox Native Americans. Caitlin's sketch was done in 1 872.The past of sexuality and the manifestation of gender differed greatly among the numerous Indigenous communities spread across the globe. Cross-gender roles, known as berdaches, were practiced in pre-colonial times by the Kaska people of the Yukon Territory, the Klamath people of southern Oregon, and the Mohave, Cocopa, and Maricopa people of the Colorado River. [3] Berdache individuals participated in the traditional roles of the other sex, including their mannerisms and labor. Cross-gender females in the Mohave tribe conducted ceremonies in which they would fully berdache females as males, giving them the right to marry women. [3] The term berdache is considered archaic in the modern era, and it has been replaced in common usage by the term 'two spirit,' which emphasizes how Native Americans themselves viewed these individuals. When it came to the majority of Native Americans, a person's spirit was more important than their physical body. They believed that a person who transgressed from their original gender took on a third gender that was distinct from either the male or female gender. [4] Two spirit natives would frequently be a part of same-sex relationships because they would fulfill the necessary responsibilities of a family unit that was expected in Native societies. [4] However, two spirit individuals of the same sex did not marry one The many different tribes each had their own unique conceptions of what marriage entailed. For example, the Navajo people practiced polygamy, and their customs required that the wives be related to each other or members of the same clan. [5] This practice was outlawed in July 1945 by the Navajo Tribal Council in response to pressure from the United States Government, which sought to put an end to the practice as it enacted its own prohibitions on polygamy. [6] Polygamy is illegal in the United States.

- Asia: India

- Article primary: a history of sexuality in India

- Additional information can be found in the Kama Sutra.

- Additional information can be found at:

- Apsarases as shown in the architecture of the Khajuraho temple

- A flying penis and a flying vulva are having sexual relations. Painting done in gouache

In ancient times, India was the origin of the philosophical focus that new-age groups use to frame their perspectives on sexuality. In modern times, India continues to play an important role in the history of sex, from the production of one of the first literatures that regarded sexual intercourse as a science to being the origin of the philosophical focus that new-age groups use to frame their perspectives on sexuality. One may make the case that India was an innovator in the field of sexual education by employing the arts and literature. In India, as in many other countries, there was a disparity in sexual habits between common people and powerful rulers, with those in power frequently indulging in hedonistic lifestyles that were not typical of general moral attitudes. Common people, on the other hand, adhered to sexual norms that were more in line with those of other societies. India is the birthplace of many of the sexual activities that are prevalent (and not so common) in the globe today. These traditions, such as the custom and art of kissing, spread to other parts of the world during the early stages of globalization.

The Kama Sutra depicted as a painting.

The earliest evidence of attitudes regarding sexuality may be found in the ancient scriptures of Hinduism, Buddhism, and Jainism. The earliest of these works are among the world's oldest pieces of literature that are still in existence today. The Vedas, which are among of the world's oldest literature, include ethical discussions of sexuality, marriage, and prayers for fertile children. It is clear that the Asvamedha Yajna was a fertility rite intended to protect and increase the kingdom's productive capacity as well as its military prowess. Sex magic was incorporated into a number of different Vedic rituals, the most significant of which was the Asvamedha Yajna. The ritual culminated with the chief queen lying with the dead horse in a simulated sexual act. The epics of ancient India, the Ramayana and the Mahabharata, which may have been written for the first time as early as 1400 BCE, had a significant impact on the culture of Asia, particularly on the culture of following generations of Chinese, Japanese, Tibetan, and South East Asian peoples. The existence of these texts lends credence to the theory that in ancient India, sexual activity was regarded as a duty shared by a married couple. According to this theory, the husband and wife took equal pleasure in one another's company during sexual encounters. However, sexual activity was regarded as a private matter by adherents of the Indian faiths listed above. It would appear that ancient societies condoned the practice of polygamy. In actuality, it appears that only the ruling classes engaged in this behavior, while the common people continued to practice monogamous marriage.

In many different societies, it is typical for the ruling elite to engage in polygamous relationships in order to ensure the continuation of the family dynasty.

The Kama Sutra depicted as a painting.

The texts of the Kama Sutra are probably the most well-known pieces of sexual literature to come out of India. These works were produced for persons who belonged to the philosopher, warrior, and nobility castes, as well as their servants and concubines, as well as those who were members of particular religious groups. These were folks who could not only read and write but also had prior experience being instructed and educated. India is the birthplace of sixty-four different arts that focus on love, passion, and pleasure. There are numerous variations of the arts that originated in Sanskrit and were later translated into other languages such as Persian or Tibetan. These variations can be found all across the world. There are many of the original documents that have been lost, and the only evidence that points to their existence can be found in other texts. One of the most famous versions of the Kama Sutra, authored by Vatsyayana, was initially rendered in English by Sir Richard Burton and F. This version of the Kama Sutra is considered to be one of the surviving texts. Arbuthnot, Francis. At this point in time, the Kama Sutra is perhaps the non-religious work that is read the most frequently all across the world. Within the context of a committed partnership, it describes the various ways in which partners can bring pleasure to one another.

- Sculpture originating from one of the temples in Khajuraho

- Cave paintings from the Ajanta region

When cultures from the Islamic world and the Victorian age of England arrived in India, they generally had a negative impact on the sexual liberty that existed in India at the time. In the context of the Indian religions, also known as dharmas, such as Hinduism, Buddhism, Jainism, and Sikhism, sex is generally either seen as a moral duty of each partner in a long term marriage relationship to the other, or it is seen as a desire that hinders spiritual detachment, and therefore must be renounced. A renaissance of sexual liberalism has taken place among the educated urban population of modern India; however, there is still discrimination, and forced marriage is still performed among the poor (forced marriage exists along a broad continuum of coercion, and the boundary between forced marriage and arranged marriage is not always agreed upon, even in the present-day context of the 2011 Istanbul Convention or the 2013 United Nations Human Rights Council resolution r). In modern India, a renaissance of sexual liberalism

Fresco frescoes that were painted inside the Ajanta caves

There are several systems of thought within Indian philosophy, such as Tantra, that place a significant emphasis on sexual activity as either a sacred duty or even as a way to attaining spiritual enlightenment or yogic equilibrium. Tantric practices can take many different forms, but the one that is most easily identifiable as left-hand Tantra is the one that involves actual sexual encounters. It is a common misconception that "Tantric sex" must always be slow and sustained, and it is possible for it to culminate in an orgasm. For instance, "there should be vigorous copulation" is a requirement according to the Yoni Tantra. Tantra, on the other hand, is unanimous in its assertion that there existed certain types of people whose personalities were incompatible with particular practices. Tantra was personality-specific, and its adherents insisted that people with pashu-bhava (animal disposition), also known as people whose natures are dishonest, promiscuous, greedy, or violent, and who consumed meat and indulged in intoxication, would only incur bad karma by following Tantric paths without the assistance of a Guru who could instruct them on the correct path. Ejaculating in front of other people is considered highly inappropriate in Buddhist tantra due to the fact that the primary objective of sexual practice is to direct one's sexual energy toward the accomplishment of full enlightenment rather than the simple pursuit of pleasure. Tantra is a philosophical system that emphasizes the importance of sensual experiences, including sexual ones.

On display are sexually explicit paintings from an album that is currently being viewed. A work of art. It is believed to date back to the late 17th century. In the middle to late 18th century, these sexually explicit paintings were displayed in pornographic albums. The I Ching, also known as "The Book of Changes," is an ancient Chinese work that deals with divination. One of the two main models that are utilized to explain the world in this text is sexual interplay. Heaven is depicted as engaging in sexual activity with Earth in a straightforward manner, without any shame or need for circumlocution. In a similar vein, the male lovers of early Chinese men of great political power are mentioned in one of the earliest great works of philosophy and literature called the Zhuang Zi (or Chuang Tzu, as it is written in the old method of romanization). This is not done out of any feeling of prurient fascination; rather, it is done with a sense of historical accuracy.

Observation of anal sexual activity between two males. Dynasty of the Qing

Sexism has a long and troubled history in China, dating back to the time of moral leaders like Confucius, who offered severely derogatory descriptions of the natural qualities that women possessed. Since ancient times, family and community have had a strong influence on whether or not a woman keeps her virginity, and this influence has been tied to the monetary value of women as a form of commodity (the "sale" of women involved the delivery of a bride price). Because of an obvious double standard, men were shielded from the consequences of their own sexual exploits. If a man had any kind of social rank in traditional society, it was almost definitely his father and/or grandpa who chose his first bride for him. However, that same guy may subsequently arrange for himself more desirable sexual companions who had the status of concubines. Concubines were sexual partners who were considered subordinate to the husband. In addition to that, the bondservants that he had in his hands might possibly have been sexually available to him. It stands to reason that not all men have the financial means to pamper themselves to such a large extent.

Three pages from an erotic album that was written in Chinese. Between the years 1701 and 1900?

It is speculated that this picture is a preliminary drawing for a painting. It is believed that the picture was made during the pre-Song period, which lasted from 960 BCE to 960 CE. It is believed that this sketch was drawn sometime between the early and middle of the 19th century. In summary, all of the features of conduct that are associated with sexuality in the West are represented in Chinese literature, including displays of affection, marital joy, unrestrained sexuality, romance, romantic dalliances, and homosexual relationships. This interest can be traced back over a long period of time. Besides the previously mentioned Zhuang Zi passages, sexuality is exhibited in other works of literature such as the Tang dynasty Yingying zhuan (Biography of Cui Yingying), the Qing dynasty Fu sheng liu ji (Six Chapters of a Floating Life), the humorous and intentionally salacious Jin Ping Mei, and the multi-faceted and insightful Hong lou meng (Dream of the Red Chamber, also called Story of the Stone). Only one of these narratives, the one about Yingying and her de facto spouse Zhang, does not detail either homosexual or heterosexual relations between the characters. The novel "Rou bu tuan," which translates to "Prayer mat of flesh," discusses even the practice of organ transplantation between other species in order to improve one's sexual performance. The Taoist classics are considered part of the canon of Chinese literature. [7] The Taoist school of thought, which is a philosophical tradition in China, is responsible for the establishment of Taoist Sexual Practices, which have three primary objectives: health, longevity, and spiritual development.

A work of art. This is Wang Sheng. Before the year 1645

A desire for respectability and the belief that all aspects of human behavior could be brought under government control have until recently mandated that official Chinese spokesmen maintain the fiction of sexual fidelity in marriage, the absence of any great frequency of premarital sexual intercourse, and the total absence in China of the so-called "decadent capitalist phenomenon" of homosexuality. This has changed recently, but until recently, official Chinese spokesmen were required to do so. It was extremely difficult for the Chinese government to take effective action against sexually transmitted illnesses, especially AIDS, until very recently as a direct result of the ideological demands that prevented objective scrutiny of sexual conduct in China. These demands existed in China until very recently. At the same time, major migrations to the cities, China's gender imbalance, and considerable levels of unemployment have led to a rebirth of prostitution in uncontrolled venues. This is a crucial factor that accelerates the spread of sexually transmitted diseases to a large number of people of the general population. In the past few decades, the influence that families have had over individuals has diminished, which has made it easier for younger generations of both men and women to find sexual and/or marital partners on their own accord. A Kabuki performer who also works as a sex worker enjoys playing with his customer while also taking advantage of the services provided by the serving girl. Shunga-style woodblock print with ink on paper depicting Nishikawa Sukenobu during the Kyoho period (1716–1735).

The primary article on the subject of sexuality in Japan

Eroticism is shown as a vital component of the aesthetic life of the nobles in the Genji Monogatari (Tale of Genji), which was written in Japan about the eighth century AD and is frequently referred to be the first novel written anywhere in the world. It is made clear that sexuality was a highly valued aspect of cultured life by the fact that Prince Genji's sexual encounters are discussed at length, in an objective manner, and in a manner that gives the impression that sexuality was treated with the same respect as music or any of the arts. Although the majority of Genji's sexual encounters are with women, there is one event that reveals a great deal about him. In this episode, Genji drives quite a distance to see one of the women with whom he occasionally consorts, but he finds that she is not at her home. Due to the late hour and the fact that sexual encounters have already been planned for the day, Genji takes pleasure in the fact that the lady's younger brother is available. According to Genji, the younger brother is equally satisfactory as an erotic partner.

Since that time and continuing at least until the Meiji Reformation, there is no evidence to suggest that sexuality was considered in a derogatory manner in any time period. In modern times, homosexuality was driven out of sight until it reemerged in the wake of the sexual revolution with seemingly little or no need for a period of acceleration. This was the first time that homosexuality was visible in contemporary times since it was forced out of sight in modern times. Yukio Mishima, who is probably the most well-known Japanese writer in the rest of the world, regularly wrote about homosexuality and the relationship that it has with both traditional and modern aspects of Japanese culture. In a similar vein, activities such as prostitution, pornography, the practice of the geisha, and a plethora of fetish and sadomasochistic subcultures have reemerged after being hidden for several decades.

In Japan, sexuality was governed by the same social factors that give Japan's culture its very distinct identity in comparison to the cultures of China, Korea, India, and Europe. Ostracism is the major tool that is utilized in Japanese society as a means of maintaining social order and maintaining social control. When it comes to determining what acts might make a person appear "corrupt" or "guilty," in the Christian sense of such words, less focus is placed on what is pleasant or proper to show other people and more on what should be done. This tendency of people in Japanese society to group in terms of "in groups" and "out groups" is a residue of Japan's long history as a caste society, and it is a source of great pressure on every facet of Japanese society, including pop culture (which is reflected in the tribal, often materialistic, and very complex nature of teenage subcultures), as well as more traditional standards (such as the high-pressure role of the salaryman). There is a wide spectrum of attitudes toward sexual expression, which goes from an absolute must to a stern no-no. As a result, many people, especially adolescents, discover that they have to play a variety of roles that are otherwise very distinct during the week.

The institution of the geisha is a frequent source of misunderstandings in relation to the sexuality of the Japanese people. A geisha was not a prostitute but rather a lady who was trained in the arts such as music and sophisticated conversation and who was available for encounters with her male clientele that were not sexual in nature. Geishas were in demand in Japan. Because, with the exception of the geisha, women were typically not expected to be prepared for anything other than the discharge of domestic responsibilities, these women were distinct from the wives that their customers probably had at home. Geisha were the only exception to this rule. This restriction, which was imposed on the majority of women in traditional society due to the usual social function that they were expected to play, resulted in a decline in the activities that those women were able to enjoy, but it also caused a limitation in the ways in which a man could enjoy the company of his wife. Geisha were handsomely compensated for their services because they were able to perform non-sexual social duties that regular women were prohibited from performing at the time. Geisha also performed sexual roles. The geisha were not deprived of opportunity to express themselves sexually or in any other seductive fashion that was appropriate given their position. It was possible for a geisha to have a patron with whom she enjoyed sexual intimacy; however, this sexual function was not part of a geisha's job or responsibility in her position as a geisha.

On the most basic level, in traditional Japanese society, women were supposed to be extremely obedient to men, and particularly to their husbands. This was especially the case in the household. Therefore, according to a socionormal assessment of their responsibilities, they were essentially little more than housekeepers and devoted sexual partners to their husbands. Their husbands, on the other hand, could sexually consort with whoever they chose outside of the family, and a major part of male social behavior involves after-work forays to places of entertainment in the company of male cohorts from the workplace — places that could easily offer possibilities of sexual satisfaction outside of the family. In addition, their wives could be unaware of their husbands' sexual relationships with other people outside of the family. This aspect of Japanese society has undergone some degree of liberalization in the postwar period in regard to the standards that were imposed on women, in addition to an extension of the de facto powers of women in the home and in the community, both of which existed unrecognized in traditional Japanese society. Since people first became aware of the AIDS epidemic, Japan has not suffered from the high rates of sickness and death that define, for example, some nations in Africa, some nations in Southeast Asia, etc. In the years since people first became aware of the AIDS epidemic, Japan has not suffered from the high rates of disease and death that characterize these other nations. As of 2004, condoms accounted for 80% of birth control use in Japan, and this may explain why Japan has comparably lower rates of AIDS than other countries[9]. In 1992, the government of Japan justified its continued refusal to allow oral contraceptives to be distributed in Japan on the fear that it would lead to reduced condom use, and thus increase the transmission of AIDS.

- Antiquity in its classical form

- A man gives his much younger sweetheart a passionate kiss on top of a cup. Approximately 480 BC

There are no citations for any sources in this section. Please contribute to the improvement of this section by adding citations to sources that can be trusted. Content that lacks appropriate citations may be contested and removed. (This message was initially published in November 2010; find out how and why it was removed)

Greco-Roman antiquity

Inscription of a sexually suggestive picture on an ancient Greek jewel Please also visit the following related articles: Homosexuality in ancient Greece, Prostitution in Ancient Greece, and Pederasty in Ancient Greece. In ancient Greece, the phallus was an object of worship as a sign of fertility. The phallus was frequently fashioned into the form of a herma. This is reflected in the sculpture of ancient Greece as well as other artworks. One view held by men in ancient Greece on the sexuality of women was that they resented the penises of men. Wives were seen as both a commodity and an instrument for the production of lawful offspring at the time. In their own households, they were forced to engage in sexual competition with eromenoi, hetaeras, and slaves.

It was Oinochoe. The artist known as Shuvalov. In the vicinity of 430–420 BCE

Both homosexuality and bisexuality, in the form of ephebophilia (which can be compared to slavery in certain aspects), were societal institutions in ancient Greece. These sexual orientations were also an important part of the country's education system, art scene, religious practices, and political structure. Adults could have romantic relationships, but society generally frowned upon this practice. Even the lesbian relationships had a paternalistic undertone to them. The interior of the box mirror container has an engraved design on the surface that has been silvered. Ancient Greek language. Located in Boston, the Museum of Fine Arts. Between the years 340 and 320 BCE

A bronze relief is embossed on the exterior of the box mirror container's casing. Ancient Greek language. Located in Boston, the Museum of Fine Arts. Approximately 340 to 320 Ancient Greek males held the view that refined prostitution was required for pleasure, and there were many distinct grades of prostitutes accessible at the time. Peripatetic prostitutes solicited business on the streets, whereas temple or consecrated prostitutes paid a higher price. Hetaera, companions who were educated and intelligent, were for intellectual as well as physical pleasure. The temple at the city of Corinth, which is located on the Aegean Sea, was home to one thousand prostitutes who had been dedicated to the gods. Anal sex is sexual activity between two males. The person seen on the left is having fun with a hula hoop. The amphora. Etruscan language. During the 5th century BCE It was common for men to commit rape, and most of the time it occurred in the context of combat. Men viewed it as their "right of dominance." Even in religious texts, rape in the sense of "abduction" followed by consensual lovemaking is depicted: Zeus is claimed to have ravaged numerous women, including Leda while she was disguised as a swan, Dana when she was dressed as golden rain, and Alkmene while she was dressed as her own husband. In another version of the myth, Zeus is shown as having raped a young boy named Ganymede.

The region of Etruria

When compared to the other ancient peoples of Europe, most of whom had inherited the Indo-European traditions and views on the gender roles, the ancient Etruscans had significantly different perspectives on sexuality than the other ancient Europeans. The Etruscans were referred to as "immoral" by Greek authors such as Theopompus and Plato. Based on their descriptions, we can deduce that it was common practice for Etruscan women to have sexual relations with men who were not their husbands, and that in Etruscan culture, children were not considered "illegitimate" simply because their parents did not know who the father was. Theopompus also mentioned orgiastic ceremonies, but it is unclear whether or not they were typical practices or whether they were merely a small ceremony performed in honor of a particular deity.

- Rome in its heyday

- A sexual encounter between a man and a woman in erotica. Pompeiian wall painting from the first century.

- Wall fresco from Pompeii depicts the "woman riding" position, a favorite in Roman art: even in vivid sex scenes, the woman's breasts are sometimes hidden by clothing or other objects.

- The following articles serve as primary sources: Homosexuality in ancient Rome, Prostitution in Ancient Rome, and Sexuality in Ancient Rome.

- Roman Spintria tokens featured explicit sexual imagery. Glasgow's Hunterian Museum and Art Gallery is a great place to visit. 22 CE until 37 CE approximately

In the Roman Republic, the concept of male sexuality was predicated on the citizen's obligation to maintain control over his own body[11]. "Virtue" (virtus, derived from the Latin word for "man") was considered synonymous with "manliness." Female sexuality was encouraged within the context of marriage. Pudicitia was the corresponding virtue for female citizens of good social standing. Pudicitia was a form of sexual integrity that exhibited their attractiveness and self-control. In Roman patriarchal society, a "real man" was intended to rule both himself and others properly, and he should not yield to the use or pleasure of others. [13] Same-sex acts were not regarded as degrading a Roman's masculinity, as long as he performed the penetrative or dominant role. Prostitutes, entertainers, and slaves were examples of acceptable male partners in this society. Other acceptable male partners include slaves. It was against the law to have sexual relations with freeborn male minors (see Lex Scantinia). The terms "homosexual" and "heterosexual" did not, therefore, form the major divide in Roman thought regarding sexuality, and there are no Latin words for either of these conceptions. [14]

- It was Cunnilingus. A painting on the wall. Baths in the suburbs of Pompeii.

- Cunnilingus, fellatio, and anal sex between two females and two males. Cunnilingus between two females and two males. Wall painting, bathrooms in the suburbs. I. Pompeii.

- a female having sexual encounters with two males. A painting on the wall. Baths in the suburbs of Pompeii.

Roman literature and art are full of explicit depictions of sexuality in both public and private settings. A common kind of ornamentation was the fascinum, which was a phallic charm. In the wall paintings that have been saved from Pompeii and Herculaneum, sexual positions and scenarios are shown in a wide variety of different ways. The Augustan poet Ovid wrote a collection of poetry called "The Art of Love," in which he satirically taught both men and women on how to seduce and pleasure lovers. These collections of poetry praised love encounters. Thinkers like Lucretius and Seneca developed elaborate ideas of human sexuality that were based on Greek philosophy. These theories were very complex. Several sexual topics, including gender identity, adultery, incest, and even rape, are frequently discussed in classical myths

Traditional Roman religion, both the public cult of the state and private religious practices and magic, supported and regulated Roman sexuality. [16] Cicero held that the desire to procreate (libido) was "the seedbed of the republic," as it was the cause for the first form of social institution, marriage, which in turn created the family, which the Romans regarded as the building block of civilization. [17] Roman law penalized sex crimes (statism), which was a violation of Adultery was only considered to have been committed by a Roman husband in the event that his sexual companion was another married lady. It was common practice, open to the public, and prostitution was legal. Gladiators were considered to have a sexual allure, and it was common practice to presume that entertainers of either gender were sexually available (see infamia). Slaves did not have legal personality, hence they were open to sexual exploitation by their masters. Anxieties about the loss of liberty and the subordination of the citizen to the emperor were expressed by a perceived increase in passive homosexual behavior among free men. [18] Sexual conquest was a frequent metaphor for Roman imperialism. [20] Anxieties about the loss of liberty and the subordination of the citizen to the emperor were expressed by a perceived increase in passive homosexual behavior among free men.

Polynésie française

There has been a lot of attention paid to the sexual culture of the Islands. The local society approves of certain sexual behaviors that are frowned upon in western civilizations and considers others to be inappropriate. Reading antique manuscripts is the only way to explore their pre-Western social history because so many of these customs have been altered as a result of contact with Western societies. Children were had to share bedrooms with their parents and were therefore able to observe their parents engaging in sexual activity. As soon as boys were physically able to do so, simulations of sexual encounters gave way to actual penetration. The adults laughed at the children's attempts to simulate sexual activity. As youngsters got closer to the age of 11, their perceptions regarding girls began to change. Incest, exogamy regulations, and firstborn daughters of high-ranking lineages were some of the factors that contributed to the suppression of adolescent libido. However, premarital sexual activity was tolerated regardless of whether or not it was encouraged. It was acceptable for high-ranking women to have extramarital affairs after the birth of their first child. The following morning, as soon as it became light, we were encircled by an even bigger crowd of these folks than the day before. At this point, there were at least one hundred different women, and all of them were trying to get on board by engaging in sexually suggestive behavior and expressions. It was not easy for me to convince my staff to follow the instructions that I had given them on this matter. There were at least a few young women in this group who were not quite ten years old. But it appears that young is not a test of innocence in this case; these children, or infants if I may call them that, rivaled their mothers in the wantonness of their movements and the skills of allurement.

Yuri Lisyansky, from his autobiography

According to Adam Johann von Krusenstern's book[24] around the same trip as Yuri's, a father sent a girl between the ages of 10 and 12 on his ship, and she had sex with the crew. Yuri's expedition was one of these expeditions. According to the book[25] written by Charles Pierre Claret de Fleurieu and Étienne Marchand, girls as young as eight years old engaged in sexual behaviors in public, including having sex and performing other sexual acts.

The 20th century: the shift in sexual mores

In the 1960s and early 1970s, the Western world underwent a significant shift in terms of sexual morality and sexual behavior as a result of what is known as the "second sexual revolution." The development of innovative and effective methods for the individual's control over whether or not they are able to become pregnant was one factor that contributed to the shift in values that were associated with sexual behaviors. Topping the list at the time was the introduction of the first oral contraceptive pill. [26] At the same time, the liberalization of abortion laws in many countries made it feasible to terminate an undesired pregnancy in a safe and legal manner, without the need to provide evidence that the birth would be extremely hazardous to the mother's health. [27]

- A warm embrace from Shah Abbas I for his wine boy. Muhammad Qasim created this painting in 1627. Louvre, located in Paris.

- Relations between people of the same gender

- The primary article on the subject: the history of homosexuality

- The lesbian sexual scene. A painting on the wall. Baths in the suburbs of Pompeii.

- Anal sex is sexual activity between two males. On paper painted with gouache. Painting by a Safavid artist. The Kinsey Institute Gallery was established in 1660.

Throughout history, societies have held a variety of views regarding same-sex relationships. These views have ranged from requiring all males to participate in same-sex relationships to casual integration to acceptance to viewing the practice as a minor sin to repressing it through law enforcement and judicial mechanisms to outlawing it under the penalty of death. "strong disapproval of homosexuality was reported for 41% of 42 cultures; it was accepted or ignored by 21%, and 12% reported no such concept," according to a comprehensive compilation of historical and ethnographic materials of pre-industrial cultures. Of 70 ethnographies, 59% reported homosexuality absent or rare in frequency, while 41% reported that it was present or not uncommon. [28] In addition, 12% reported that there was no such concept. In societies that were inspired by Abrahamic religions, the law and the church codified sodomy as a violation of divine law or a crime committed against nature. However, the concept that anal intercourse between males should be forbidden predates the Christian religion. It was common practice in ancient Greece, and the term "unnatural" can be dated back to Plato[29]. Many historical figures, including Socrates, Lord Byron, Edward II, and Hadrian,[30] have had terms such as gay or bisexual applied to them. Some academics, such as Michel Foucault, have regarded this as risking the anachronistic introduction of a contemporary construction of sexuality that is foreign to their times, though others challenge this notion. The contention that no one in antiquity or the middle ages experienced homosexuality as an exclusive, permanent, or defining way of sexuality is a recurring thread running through constructionist arguments. John Boswell has provided a rebuttal to this argument by referring to ancient Greek literature penned by Plato[35] that depict people who demonstrate exclusive homosexualitThe intersection of religion and sex

- Article principal: sexuality and religious belief

- Religions based on Abraham

Abrahamic religions (including Judaism, Samaritanism, Christianity, the Baha'i Faith, and Islam) have traditionally affirmed and endorsed a patriarchal and heteronormative approach towards human sexuality. These religions favor exclusively penetrative vaginal intercourse between men and women within the boundaries of marriage over all other forms of human sexual activity,[38] including auto-eroticism, masturbation

Jewish religion

When sexual activity takes place within the context of a marriage, Jewish law does not view it as inherently immoral or humiliating, nor does it view it as a necessary evil for the goal of procreation. It is generally accepted that sexual activity between a married couple should be kept secret and sanctified. The following list of sexually deviant behaviors was once regarded as "abominations" due to its extreme immorality and was often deemed a capital offense punishable by death. Ablution was necessary whenever there was sexual residue outside of the body since it was regarded ritually impure.

However, rabbinic Judaism had unequivocally condemned homosexuality. Recently, some academics have questioned whether the Old Testament forbade all types of homosexuality, noting concerns of translation and references to ancient cultural norms. [54] However, rabbinic Judaism had condemned homosexuality. And God blessed them, and God said to them, "Be fruitful and multiply, and fill the earth and subdue it, and rule over the fish of the sea and over the fowl of the sky and over all the beasts that tread upon the earth." (Genesis 1:28) This passage is taken from Genesis 1:28. Adultery, all types of incest, male homosexuality, bestiality, and the introduction of the idea that one should not have sex while their wife is having her period are all examples of partnerships that are forbidden by the Torah, despite the fact that the Torah is fairly forthright in its depiction of various sexual practices.

- You are not allowed to have sexual relations with the wife of your neighbor or you will be ritually impure (Lev. 18:20).

- It is an abomination for you to lay with humanity, just as it is an abomination for womankind (Lev. 18:22).

And you shall have no sexual relations with any animal, lest you become polluted by it; and a woman shall not approach an animal with the intention of having sexual relations with it; this is immorality (Lev. 18:23). And during the uncleanness of a woman's separation from her husband, you are not allowed to approach her in order to reveal her nakedness (Lev. 18:19). The original meanings of these lines have not changed, but their interpretation may have altered when they were translated into English and other languages. This view, however, has been counteracted by conservatives. The above sections may, however, be open to modern interpretation.

The Christian faith

Christianity re-emphasised the Jewish attitudes on sexuality by adding two new concepts. First, there was the re-iterated idea that marriage was absolutely exclusive and indissoluble. This placed further guidance on divorce and expanded on the reasons and principles behind those laws. Second, in Old Testament times, marriage was almost universal, in continuity with the total matrimony in Eden. However, in the New Testament, the trajectory is extended forward to the goal of no marriage at all. Paul, in one of his letters to the church in Corinth, specifically answers several issues that members of that congregation had raised about the norms governing sexual interactions. The New Testament is very explicit on these concepts.

1 Now concerning the matters about which you wrote, 'It is well for a man not to touch a woman.' 2 However, because of cases of sexual immorality, each man should have his own wife and each woman should have her own husband. 3 The husband should give to his wife her conjugal rights, and likewise the wife should give to her husband. 4 For the wife does not have authority over her own body, but the husband does; and similarly, the husband does not have authority over his own body, but Paul is speaking into a situation in which the church was slipping into desire, and some members were even employing prostitutes (6:16). At the same time, others preached a 'higher spirituality' that incorrectly denied pleasure from worldly things, including abstention from sex (7:1). Paul is preaching into this situation. Paul writes to them to explain the appropriate setting for sexual activity within marriage, as well as the significance of partners continuing to engage in sexual activity and give each other pleasure. However, he also encourages them to pursue celibacy in those situations where God has given them the ability to do so (7:7), so that they can devote more of their time and energy to serving the needs of others.

There are a number of other texts that discuss sexual activity or marriage. Augustine of Hippo was of the opinion that prior to Adam's fall, the sexual act was fully subject to human reason and that there was no such thing as lust involved in it. Later theologians came to the same conclusion, which was that the lust that is associated with sexuality is a product of original sin. However, almost all of them came to the conclusion that this was only a venial sin provided it was conducted within the context of a marriage and did not include excessive lust. In Reformed educational institutions, such as those based on the Westminster Confession as an example, there is an emphasis placed on the following three reasons why people get married: to promote mutual encouragement, support, and pleasure; to have children; and to avoid lustful sin. The concept that there is no guilt at all in the unrestricted enjoying of marital intercourse has gained traction among a significant number of Christians in modern times. Some Christians have a tendency to restrict the situations and the extent to which sexual pleasure is ethically acceptable. This may be done for a variety of reasons, including the development of self-control to prevent sex from becoming addictive or as a form of fasting.

Islam (faith)

Only after marriage is sexual intercourse permitted in Islam; however, it is not regarded as inherently evil or shameful when it is carried out within the context of a marriage. Some forms of sexual deviance are regarded as "abominations" due to their grave lack of morality and are occasionally subject to the death penalty. After engaging in sexual activity, one must first undergo a full-body cleansing before beginning to pray. Such extra-marital intercourse, referred to as zina in the Qur'an, is punishable in few countries that fully practice Islamic law (Sharia) by corporal punishment of 100 lashes if the person is unmarried (fornication) and by death if the person is married to another (adultery). If a Muslim engaged in sexual intercourse with anyone other than the spouse, then this would be considered sinful, as well as a crime. This is only the case if the actual act of copulation was witnessed by four persons who will testify to such, and according to the text of the Qur'an, the punishment for bringing unfounded charges is eighty lashes if the accuser cannot present four witnesses to testify to the act. In most cases, this indicates that the perpetrators of the wrongdoing do not face the consequences for their actions unless they admit their guilt on four separate occasions and, as a result, become liable to be penalized for the offense.

Religions based on Dharma

There are no citations for any sources in this section. Please contribute to the improvement of this section by adding citations to sources that can be trusted. Content that lacks appropriate citations may be contested and removed. (January 2013) (Find out when this template message can be removed and how to do so)

In India, Hinduism encouraged an open and accepting approach towards sexuality in all of its forms, including as an art, a science, and a spiritual practice. The Kamasutra (Aphorisms on Love) and the Kamashastra (from Kama, which means pleasure, and shastra, which means specialized knowledge or method) are two of the most well-known works of Indian literature pertaining to sexuality. This compilation of explicit sexual literature, which include both spiritual and practical advice, covers the vast majority of topics pertaining to human courting and sexual encounters. The sage Vatsyayana took a manuscript containing 150 chapters, which had been condensed from 300 chapters, which had been derived from a compilation including over 100,000 chapters of literature, and put it all together in its current form. Based on the material that has been found that is circumstantial, it is believed that the Kamasutra was written in its final form sometime between the third and fifth century AD. The sculptures that were carved on the temples in India, particularly the ones at the Khajuraho temple, are also famous. The forthright depiction of unconstrained sex provides a glimpse into a more liberated culture and a time when people believed in dealing openly with all areas of life. This provides a peek at the emancipated society. On the other hand, there is a school of thought that maintains that the presence of sexually suggestive carvings outside of temples is a sign that visitors should enter the temples with no desires (kama) in their hearts.

- In addition to Vatsyayana's Kamashastra, which is without a doubt the most well-known of all of these kinds of works, there are a number of other volumes, such as the following:

- The Ratirahasya, whose name literally translates to "the secrets of love" (rahasya) is also known as "the union of love."

- The Panchasakya, also known as the five arrows (sakya);

- The Ratimanjari, also known as the "Garland of Love" (manjari) or "the Union of Love" (rati).

- The stage of love, also known as the Ananga Ranga.

Kukkoka is the name of the poet who penned the book "The Secrets of Love." It is thought that he wrote this book on his work in order to appease one Venudutta, who was regarded as a king at the time. It has been many years since this work was translated into Hindi. At that time, the author's name was shortened to Koka, and the book he wrote was given the title Koka Shastra. All of the translations into the many languages spoken in India ended up using the same name. The term "doctrines of love" (Kama Shastra) is synonymous with the term "doctrines of Koka," which translates directly to "doctrines of Koka." Both of these terms, "doctrines of love" and "doctrines of Koka," are used interchangeably.

Both sex and technology

Midway through the 20th century, advancements in medical research and a more contemporary understanding of the menstrual cycle led to the development of observational, surgical, chemical, and laboratory procedures. These techniques allowed for the identification and treatment of many different types of infertility. Because the idea that women could prevent pregnancy with a medication incited fear in many people due to misogynistic views on women and their roles as birth givers, the birth control pill was illegal in many countries, including the United States and Canada. The pill was introduced in the 1960s and allowed women to control if and when they had children, which increased their freedom sexually and socially. [56] The pill was illegal in many countries, including the United States and Canada. Some people believed that taking the pill made women more masculine, which led the Catholic Church to state that only married women should be able to access it. This was done so that single women would not be encouraged to engage in sexually deviant behavior. [57] In 1974, the United States Supreme Court legalized taking the pill for unmarried people with the case Eisenstadt v. Baird, and in 1978, it ruled that states cannot place any restrictions on an individual's ability to access the pill. [58]

The zoophobia

Sexual intercourse between humans and animals, often known as zoophilia or bestiality, most likely dates back to prehistoric times. Bestiality remained a common theme in mythology and folklore through the classical period and into the Middle Ages (e.g. Leda and the Swan), and several ancient authors purported to document it as a regular, accepted practice—although typically in "other" cultures. Depictions of humans and animals in a sexual context appear infrequently in rock art in Europe beginning around the beginning of the Neolithic and the domestication of animals.

The Abrahamic religions left as a legacy the explicit legal prohibition of human sexual contact with animals: the Hebrew Bible imposes the death penalty on both the person and the animal involved in an act of bestiality, and there are several examples known from medieval Europe of people and animals being executed for committing bestiality. Bestiality and other sexual "crimes against nature" were eventually incorporated into civil sodomy legislation during the Age of Enlightenment. Despite this, sodomy was typically considered a punishable offense leading to the death penalty. In the vast majority of countries, bestiality is still considered criminal. It is argued that having sex with animals is inherently abusive, despite the fact that religious and "crime against nature" arguments may still be used to justify this today. In common with many other paraphilias, the internet has allowed for the formation of a zoophile community that is beginning to lobby for zoophilia to be considered an alternative sexuality and for the legalization of bestiality.

Sexual exploitation

The exchange of monetary compensation for sexual services, such as oral sex or sexual encounters, is known as prostitution. Someone once coined the phrase "world's oldest profession" to refer to prostitution. At the very least 700 years ago, there was evidence of gonorrhea infection, which was linked to a neighborhood in Paris once known as "Le Clapiers" where prostitutes frequently operated The social class of prostitutes and the degree to which they were accepted in society was not consistent across historical eras and geographic locations. In ancient Greece, the meretrices were often women of a lesser social rank than the hetaerae, who were typically women of a higher social class. In 1988, the government of India passed a law that made it illegal for Hindu temples in south India to employ prostitutes known as Devadasi.

Diseases that are transmitted by sexual contacts transmitted sexually and safe sexual practices

Sexually transmitted illnesses have been present for a significant portion of the history of the human race. They spread throughout society unchecked until antibiotics were discovered [citation needed]. The creation of affordable condoms and education about sexually transmitted illnesses have helped to limit the danger of transmission. Due to the free movement of people and the uncontrolled distribution of antibiotics, organisms resistant to antibiotics quickly spread and, at the present time, pose a threat to people who have more than one sex partner. [Citation needed] For a period of about thirty years (during the second half of the twentieth century), their threat subsided. [Citation needed] However, due to the free movement of people and the uncontrolled distribution of antibiotics, their threat has returned.

AIDS

AIDS has had a significant impact on the sexuality of modern society. In the 1970s and 1980s, it was first discovered (although some historians claim that the first case was in 1959) spreading among gay men and those who used intravenous drugs. [Citation needed] However, some historians believe that the first case was in 1959. Due to a lack of access to medical care and educational opportunities, the majority of people who are infected with HIV today are heterosexual women, men, and children living in poor nations. The fear of catching AIDS has prompted a revolution in sex education, which now places an emphasis on the use of protection and abstinence, and also explains sexually transmitted diseases and how to prevent them. According to the BBC News, further effects of this disease run deep and have a profound impact on the expected average lifespan. "[The expected average lifespan] is falling in many African countries—a girl born today in Sierra Leone could expect to live to only 36, in contrast to Japan, where today's newborn girl might reach 85 on average."

Three

health requirements

In the course of doing a survey of the scholarly papers, books, journals, and other sources that are pertinent to a specific subject, theory, or field of research, a literature review also provides a description, summary, and critical analysis of the works that have been surveyed. The purpose of writing a literature review is to present an overview of the sources that were investigated during the process of researching a particular issue and to explain to your readers how the research fits into the greater field of study.

This chapter provides a concise survey of the literature that is currently accessible regarding the Sexual Minority community. This permits researchers to investigate the many distinct facets of the subject matter being studied. When it comes to the examination of ideas such as social exclusion, stigma, discrimination, and violations of human rights, etc..., the literature pertaining to sexual minority communities is, to a certain extent, lacking. As a result of the limited number of researchers that have investigated these subjects, there is not a vast array of published material available on the subject. The purpose of the study named "Sexual Minorities and Social Exclusion: A Study of Dharwad District in Karnataka" is to investigate the living situations of sexual minorities, as well as the factors that contribute to their social exclusion.

Exclusion, the discrimination they had to confront throughout their lives and the effects it had on them, as well as the factors that led to their social exclusion. The purpose of this chapter is to present a review of the information that is available in the literature on a variety of existential concerns faced by sexual minorities or those who identify as third gender. This chapter examines a variety of topics that are associated with sexual minorities. Some of these topics include: sexual identity; family; environment; discrimination against sexual minorities; social, political, and economic status; health concerns; violence; legal and civil rights; and human rights. Etc. The main purpose of this chapter is to provide comprehensive coverage of information that is directly linked to sexual minorities as well as information that is indirectly related to all aspects of the lives of sexual minorities. The researcher was able to identify the research gap with the help of this chapter. This chapter provides the reader with the opportunity to gain a bird's-eye view of the research that has been conducted or finished in this field up to this point. In the context of this study, relevant books, journal articles, theses, dissertations, government reports and documents, newspaper stories, guidelines from the United Nations, research websites, and other credible sources have been thoroughly examined and are given here in a logical order.

- In order to acquire a comprehensive understanding of the subject at hand, the reviews that are provided in this chapter have been broadly divided into two sections.

- Understanding Sexual Minorities and Gender Identity Variants is Covered in Part I.

This section contains a brief note on indigenous (studies done in India) and international (studies done in other countries) researches, theories, essays, and opinions of academics regarding the sexual minorities, their identities, history, and other related topics. According to the writers Berger and Luckmann (1966), sexuality is "grounded in biological drives." However, this does not define when, where, or for what reason a person engages in sexual behavior. However, sexuality is constantly channeled in definite directions socially rather than physically, which imposes restrictions on the conceptions of sexuality and renders certain forms of behavior acceptable, such as any kind of heterosexual behavior. physically, sexuality is more fluid and open to interpretation. This means that any sort of homosexual behavior is not in accordance with the social norms, and that such a group would be included in the category of sexual minorities, which includes those who are lesbian, gay, bisexual, and transgender. People who do not identify as heterosexual and belong to sexual minorities are frequently referred to as "sinful" or "deviant."

do not fit into a society that was established according to heteronormativity. This leads to antipathy toward sexual minorities, and the term most usually used to describe this hostility is "homophobia." This research was carried out in the city of Agra in India by Veena N. A. Goswami (1973). The findings of the study revealed that although the Hijras of Agra city represented two different religions—Hinduism and Islam—they all worshipped the Bahuchara Devi. The author discusses three different Hijra sects: the pure Hijras, the Randis, and the Jananas. The pure Hijras come in first place. In addition, they had the practice, which was known as Jamat, of traveling to Hijras located in various parts of India. According to the author, the majority of respondents in the survey went into the Hijra occupation freely, and very few went into the occupation when they were adolescents. The primary factors that led to them deciding to leave their native home were the fact that they had been mistreated by their parents, that they were considered Kalanka by their family, or that they had been taunted by other people. Some people were drawn to this line of work due to the fact that it allowed them to live an autonomous lifestyle and provided them with opportunities to sing and dance. Begging, singing, and dancing were the three activities that most exemplified the Hijra occupation. While the Jananas engaged in the activity of street dancing, the Randis were prostituting themselves.

The majority of the Hijras exhibited their utmost happiness through the art of singing and dancing, which brought them enormous joy. However, their biggest source of frustration was the fact that they were unable to have children. The Hijras had the belief that the ability to sing and dance was a divine gift bestowed upon them by their Devi and that it did not require any formal instruction. There was a system known as the Guru-Chela, and at the top of the hierarchy, there was one Guru known as the Mudh Guru. After the guru had died away, the Dholak was given to the Chela in accordance with his standing as the most senior practitioner in the field. When it came to the order of the activities, the Hijras placed the Randis and the Jananas lower on the totem pole than they did themselves, and vice versa. The Hijras had a fluctuating income depending on the time of year; they performed songs and dances at the birth of both boys and girls, as well as earned extra money during marriages and festivals; yet, they continued to beg throughout the year. Although some of the Hijras did engage in prostitution as a way to supplement their income or even to satiate their personal urges, they did not do so in the Guru's presence out of fear of being punished. Prostitution was practiced as a means of generating more cash. The vast majority of responders indicated that castration was not necessary in order to participate in the occupation. According to the author, the Hijras should have been granted the right to vote just like every other citizen because they were also human beings and should have been treated as such. They were told by the municipal authorities in Agra that they did not have the right to vote since they did not fit the category of either "men" or "women," and the poll workers did not know where to write their names.

Trupti Jhaveri (1989) conducted this study with the objectives of exploring the manner in which individuals enter the Hijras community; to study the religious and socio-cultural practices which influence their life; to draw up a profile of Hijras in terms of their perception of themselves physically, socially, and emotionally; to explore their conditions of living; to investigate their means of livelihood; to investigate their interaction amongst themselves; and to investigate their interaction with society; and to investigate the possibility of establishing The research came to the following conclusions: the Hijras who participated in the study had castrated themselves, either medically or traditionally, and they have done so voluntarily; the Hijras who participated in the study entered the Hijra community between the ages of 13 and 21; the study was completed. Hijras are not living with their families for one of two reasons: either the family has rejected them or they do not want to go back because it would be stigmatizing for the families to have a Hijra in the family. The family background and child rearing practices have played an important role in joining the Hijra community. Hijras are not living with their families because either the family has rejected them or they do not want to go back. At the present time, not a single Hijra is residing within the Hijra community; rather, all of the Hijras have chosen to live on their own. During their childhood, some Hijras have displayed womanly characteristics and a predisposition for roles traditionally associated with women. According to James D., et al. (1995), the United States (US) is becoming more isolated in its legal handling of sexual minorities or partnerships between people of different genders or gender identities. It is inevitable that members of sexual minorities will always have to fight a defensive battle against the perception of normalcy held by the broader public (the cis gender population). In this context, the authors propose a comparative legal analysis, which serves as an effective source of authority for domestic civil rights litigators. The authors go on to argue that in some nations sexual minorities are still at risk of being subjected to state-sanctioned murder, torture, arbitrary arrest, and other forms of human rights abuses.

In her most influential work, 'Gender Trouble,' published in 2002, Judith Butler contended that feminism had made a mistake when it tried to assert that women were a collective with common features and interests. Butler believed that women should be treated as individuals. According to the author, an unknowing regulation and reification of gender relations strengthen a view of gender relations in which human beings are divided into two distinct groups, namely men and women. Rather than opening up possibilities for a person to form and choose their own individual identity, feminism had closed down the options, and as a result, feminism had closed down the possibilities. To put it another way, Butler proposed that rather than being an immutable characteristic of a person, gender should be understood as a variable that fluctuates and changes depending on the circumstances of the situation as well as the time and place. This concept of identity belonging to

free-floating, in the sense that it is not related to an essence but rather a performance, given that this is one of the central themes in queer theory. Ulrike Boehmer (2002) conducted this study to evaluate the extent to which lesbian, gay, bisexual, and transgender (LGBT) communities have been researched in the public health research over the past twenty years. Secondary literature materials, such as papers on human subjects that were published between the years 1980 and 1999, were analyzed for this study. The study was based on these sources. The results of this study have compiled a list of all of the articles that include LGBT people. The articles were evaluated using a coding method that classified the content into various categories, such as subject matter, sexual orientation, race or ethnicity, and so on. According to the author, there were 3777 published pieces that discussed LGBT concerns (between the years 1980 and 1999). 61% of the articles focused on a particular ailment, and 85% of the articles completely ignored any mention to race or ethnicity. Studies that did not focus on sexually transmitted diseases (STDs) addressed lesbians and gay men with an equal level of frequency. On the other hand, bisexual people were given less priority in the studies, while transgender people were the subject of the least amount of research. The author concludes by stating that research on public health has ignored LGBT issues, and that there is a dearth of study on the physical and mental health of LGBT individuals.

According to the author Butler J. (2004), the term "transgender" refers to people who cross-identify or who live as another gender, but who may or may not have undergone any hormonal treatments or sex reassignment surgical operations. Among transsexuals and transgendered persons, there are some who identify as men (if female to male) or women (if male to female), and there are still others who identify as trans; as transgender, regardless of whether or not they have undergone The author further claimed that those who identify as transgendered or transsexual face discrimination and even physical assault because of their identities. According to the author Subir K Kole (2007), queerness, which refers to sexual and gender minorities, has become a problem on a global scale. On the one hand, queer mobilization and sexual identity politics are raising fundamental questions or issues like citizenship and human rights. On the other hand, discourses of nationalism, cultural identity, imperialism, tradition, and family values are being challenged. Many developing countries are currently experiencing queer mobilization and sexual identity politics. The author continues by saying that while there are some scholars who suggest that economic

Others believe that globalization is not a significant factor in global queer mobilization and sexual identity politics, despite the fact that in the developing world, a Western dominant construct of lesbian, gay, bisexual, and transgender (LGBT) identity has been exported to traditional societies, thereby destroying indigenous sexual cultures and diversities. According to Editorial (2008), Section 377 of the Indian Penal Code (IPC) should be removed since it violates the constitutional rights of sexual and gender minorities in India. According to the provisions of Section 377, those who engage in carnal intercourse "against the order of nature" shall be subject to the maximum punishment of life in prison, which can be reduced to a maximum sentence of 10 years in jail, and may also be subject to a fine. This article of the Indian Penal Code is only infrequently enforced against non-heterosexuals; however, its illegality resides in the widespread use of it by lower-level police personnel to blackmail, extort payments, and harass people in general. It is sufficient to ensure that members of sexual minorities cannot live their lives openly if they are afraid of being prosecuted. In the piece that was published in the New Statesman (2008), the author discusses Hijras. They have a history that dates back more than 4,000 years, and it has been recorded. Legends from the distant past attribute to them the ability to bestow good fortune and fertility upon others. Nevertheless, despite this presumed or believed sanctioned role in Indian culture and history, Hijras experience significant harassment and discrimination from every side. This is despite the fact that they are a minority. Nobody ever says things like, "I wish I could be a Hijra or a transgender person." A Hijra person is one who possesses the body of a man but the soul of a woman. However, this way of thinking in traditional Indian culture is starting to shift, and at the moment there appears to be both subtle and appreciable shifts taking place in terms of how these groups are being treated and recognized by mainstream society.

The author Geetanjali Misra (2009) investigated the successful struggle against a provision in section 377 of the Indian Penal Code that criminalized private consensual sex between adults of the same sex. Geetanjali Misra's research was published in 2009. People participating in gay activities (same sex) were exposed to frequent beatings and blackmail attempts by police officers, who used the threat of punishment against them. This was a direct result of Section 377 of the Indian Penal Code, which had led to considerable prejudice against people engaging in homosexual activities. In addition, non-governmental organizations that work with sexual and gender minorities have been subject to harassment and, in some cases, criminal charges under section 377 of the Indian Penal Code. This statute, which stigmatizes homosexuality and threatens gender minorities with incarceration, is believed to have slowed the progress of gay rights in India.

fight against HIV/AIDS in its various forms. After a creative and ongoing effort in the mainstream media, the clause was amended in July of 2009 to make it less restrictive. Voices Against Section 377 brought together previously marginalized sexuality and lesbian, gay, bisexual, and transgender (LGBT) individuals, as well as groups working in the areas such as children's rights and feminist groups, demonstrating that support for non-discrimination towards sexual minorities was widespread. In addition, for sexual and gender minorities to achieve complete acceptance and equality within Indian society, adjustments in both the law and society are desperately required. However, the verdict of the court of law went beyond the LGBT issue by implying protection for all sexual and gender minorities. It also presented the concept of sexual citizenship to South Asia for the very first time. According to the authors of the Mani et al. (2009) study, in modern parlance, the term "transgender" functions as an umbrella term. In India, those who identify as transgender are referred to as Hijaras, Kinnars, and Aravanies, depending on where they are located around the country. The term "transgender" refers to a broad category that encompasses a wide range of people whose behaviors and social groups frequently deviate from the conventional gender standards. There is a widely held misconception that persons of the Hijara race are neither masculine nor female. Author further says that Hijaras are socially excluded, and this social exclusion not only generates tension, violence, and disruption but also perpetuates inequality and deprivation in society. Hijaras are mostly such people who are born with male physiology and adopt feminine gender identity, women's clothing, and other feminine gender role. Hijaras are socially excluded. Author further says that Hijaras are socially excluded.

According to the research report published by the Humsafar Trust (2010), one identified risk category for HIV/AIDS in India includes men who have sex with other men (also abbreviated as MSM). This MSM community suffers many and complicated obstacles in addition to the risk of HIV infection. These challenges should be taken into account in HIV/AIDS preventive and treatment programs since they are important. There are either very few or no studies done on the mental health problems faced by MSMs in India. Stigmatization, demands from families to get married, homophobia in the community or society, crimes and criminalization, and prejudice are some of the difficulties that persons who identify as MSM must contend with. In the MSM community, these pressures can contribute to mental health problems such as sadness, anxiety, and an inclination toward suicide behavior, among other things. The author Gloria T. Di-Fulvio (2011) stated how sexual minority kids are at an elevated risk for bad health outcomes such as substance misuse, depression, anxiety, and the inclination to consider or attempt suicide. According to the author, a variety of studies have shown that

that being victimized due to one's sexual orientation is a major factor in predicting such consequences. Social connectedness, also known as the significance of belonging, which occurs when young people recognize that they are cared for and given authority within a certain setting, has been linked to favorable outcomes for young people. The life story methodology was applied in the present qualitative investigation. The life stories of individuals are generally considered to be vital representations of one's identity and are influenced by personal, social, and cultural circumstances. These contexts can be broken down into three categories: personal, social, and cultural. Twenty-two interviews with young people ranging in age from fourteen to twenty-two years old were carried out for the purpose of this study. Additionally, two focus group discussions with young people were also carried out. In the state of Massachusetts (United States), both rural and urban communities contributed youth for the recruitment effort. In addition to making a contribution to the existing body of literature on the voices of sexual minority teenagers, this research also investigates the significance of social connection in the lives of these individuals. Young people describe the manner in which interpersonal connections and group affiliations served to agree upon one's identity and offered a stage for going from personal struggle to communal efforts. The findings of this study imply that it is necessary to reconceive of the effects of disconnection (such as depression, anxiety, and the tendency to consider suicide) from individual illness and to pay attention to these affects as a response to discrimination and stigma.

According to the author Gurvinder Kalra (2011), Indian culture has always been accepting of a variety of sexual identities and sexual behaviors. This can be seen in Indian mythology and ancient books like the Kama sutra. Within Indian society, the transgendered Hijra group, also known as the transgender community, has developed over time to build a subculture that is one of a kind and distinctive from the heterosexual family. This subculture within the transgender community has traditionally kept its traditions and way of life a closely guarded secret; however, this dynamic is beginning to shift in recent years. Although there is a growing awareness regarding HIV/AIDS difficulties in the transgender community among both community members and health professionals, the same cannot be said for the issues that pertain to this community's mental health. The author of the study, Joshua Hepple (2012), discusses the development of equal rights for sexual and gender minorities by examining homosexuality and the law related to them. By looking in depth at the origins of homosexual (same sex)laws, we can understand the way in which discrimination and violence against and ill treatment of homosexuals has been justified, and many countries in recent years have and have not, repealed such homosexual (same sex) laws and promoted equal rights. It is clear that there is a great deal of diversity among the countries that surround us.

the nations of the globe with regard to the position they take on the use of criminal punishments against people whose sexual orientation is different from the conventional so-called heterosexuality. This is an old debate, but what's noteworthy is that the problems faced by homosexuals are now being framed in terms of human rights. This can give a boost to the movement for equal rights for sexual and gender minorities, which is an important development. Ina Goel et al. (2012) authors mentioned that recently the Supreme Court of India issued a notice and asked the central and all state governments why not the sexual/gender minorities or transgender should not be considered as a third sex (after male and female) and authorities should try to raise social, economic, and public health concerns towards the transgender community. In addition, the authors mentioned that the Supreme Court of India issued the notice. In this case, the questions need to be posed in a different way due to the various issues of the sexual and gender minorities as well as the transgender community. The author suggests that the question should start from an inappropriate positioning of established hierarchies in genders and suggested gender roles, already there is a struggle going on to break away from the binaries of gender (male and female), and also to set displaced trajectories to further unclear the gender constructs, which will pose serious limitations to the understanding of such a complex issue, and thus lead to further alienation of this transgender community

On the basis of the findings of the study, Dr. Venkatesan Chakrapani (2013) made several recommendations and proposals for the health and safety of Men who have sex with men (MSM), Hijras, and transgender individuals in India. Those recommendations are as follows:

• Educate and sensitize the general public as well as other stakeholders on issues pertaining to sexual and gender minorities in order to reduce the amount of social stigma and prejudice that is associated with sexual and gender minorities and to increase the level of acceptance of communities like these within mainstream society.

• As part of HIV prevention efforts undertaken by the government and other partner organizations, MSM and Hijras/Transgender individuals should be offered the opportunity to receive mental health counseling and referral services.

• Take action to reduce self-stigma among MSM and transgender individuals so that more people can embrace themselves as they are.

• Within the context of HIV prevention efforts, consider how to account for variations in condom use across various types of male partners

• Improve the social support networks of those who identify as MSM as well as Hijras and transgender people by building their communities and encouraging acceptance within their families is a priority for them.

• Take measures to lessen the discrimination that people of different sexual orientations confront in a variety of settings. places and situations

- Develop a comprehensive national health policy for sexual minorities that takes into account mental health issues.
  - Aniruddha Dutta (2013) conducted research for this study, which examined how the relationship between Indian and
  - activism for the rights of gender and sexual minorities and the action taken by the government towards it
  - According to the author, developmental organizations like the government and non-governmental organizations (NGOs) build
  - criterion for sexual orientation or gender identity that rules out participation. In addition, the author contends that,
  - The consolidation of accepted methods of readable identification is helped by such institutional ties.
  - that can justify specific gender and sexual forms of difference for the purpose of inclusion of such
  - communities within the framework of the developmental programs or activities and citizenship. But
  - the author disagrees with various alternative forms of community development which are rendered

- illegitimate as well as incomprehensible. This article also concentrates on the masculine gender that is ascribed.

- Under categories such as transgender and MSM (men), those who desire the same sex can be considered variant.

- who engage in sexual activity with guys). In addition, the transgender community is becoming increasingly globalized, which

- Providing transgender people with a type of political identification has promised them increased rights and governmental

- participation in growth-oriented initiatives for individuals with gender variant identities. The article also illustrates

- hence, a broader MSM-transgender description of identification should be founded on a

- standardization of the difference between cisgender homosexuals and male-to-female transsexuals

- persons who transition between genders.

- The authors Govindasamy Agoramoorthy et al. (2014) investigated the transgender population.

- community's former triumphs, its current challenges, and its goals for the future in the context of the

- India is the most populous democracy in the world. People who identify as transgender have been significant in the

- They played an important They were described as having a part in ancient Indian culture and tradition for over a thousand years

- in well-known religious texts and epics from the Hindu tradition, such as the Ramayana and the Mahabharata.

- Mughal kings sometimes gave transgender people key responsibilities in the royal courtyards of their palaces.

- This can be investigated further in the history of medieval India. The decline of transgender people started only

- at the beginning of the eighteenth century, when the British were first establishing their rule in India, transgender

- were excluded from society and considered to be members of the criminal underworld. That only occurred in the

- 2014 is the year that the Supreme Court of India handed down a historic decision by determining that

People who identify as transgender should be given equal chances in all aspects of society. In spite of this legal recognition, the transgender population as a whole has been compelled to live on the margins of contemporary Indian society, which means that they are not included in the majority of its activities. The authors go on to argue that because transgender people are mostly excluded from the mainstream social order, there is no data available on the mental health difficulties that transgender people confront in India. However, unfortunately, discrimination against transgender people occurs even when they seek medical aid in health care centers or hospitals. As a result, legislation that are effective in preventing discrimination against transgender people are urgently required. The question of sex-change surgery procedures is not currently being addressed by India's judicial system in any way. Therefore, the legal status of sex change surgery needs to be defined, and after that, only hospitals that are sponsored by the government should be allowed to provide subsidized health care services that are backed by competent medical surgeons. In addition, it is of the utmost need to provide proper trainings to healthcare staff on how to deal with transgender health issues. This will ensure that transgender individuals have access to high-quality medical care free from additional discrimination. Above all else, the general public in society needs to be more accepting and sympathetic toward the transgendered people of the country, and they need to treat them equally as fellow citizens so that the long-oppressed sexual and gender minority can finally be set free.

According to the Boundless (2014) research, the process of young children coming to terms with their gender identification is quite variable. It is generally accepted that it occurs between the ages of three and six years. However, many people who identify as transgender, gender queer, or gender fluid (sexual or gender minority individuals) do not have the ability to fully accept their real gender identity until much later stages of life. This is primarily because of the social stigma that is connected with these identities. According to the findings of psychological studies, children acquire their sense of gender identity in three distinct stages. In the first stage, which occurs when they are toddlers and pre-schoolers, children learn about defined characteristics, which are features of gender that are socialized. In the second stage, known as consolidation, gender identity begins to solidify somewhere between the ages of 5 and 7 years old. In the third stage, which occurs after this pinnacle of rigidity, flexibility returns along with socially determined gender roles. Times of India (2014) in an article that was published in the daily Times of India, it was said that finally there has been an official count of the third gender (sexual minorities) in the country, and that number is 4.9 lakh. Despite the fact that the census only counted persons who defined themselves as belonging to one of two genders, members of sexual minorities are ecstatic that such a big number of people described themselves

HEALTH REQUIREMENTS 141

as belonging to a third gender. Transgender activists believe that the number of people who identify as belonging to a third gender is six to seven times higher than the official count.

The counting of votes took conducted long in advance of April 2014, when the Supreme Court of India issued its order mandating the legal recognition of a third gender. Nearly 55,000 people in India are between the ages of 0 and 6 years old, according to the total count of transgender and sexual minority communities that were detected by India's census. The community of sexual minorities was taken aback by these numbers since they did not anticipate that so many parents would acknowledge that their children identify with a gender that is not male or female. In addition, the efforts of election commissions throughout the voter registration process have brought dismay to the community of sexual minorities. throughout this process, just 28,341 people were registered as belonging to a third gender. On the other hand, the information from the census represents positive news for the transgender community. However, a small number of people within the community stated that even the already known figure of 4.9 lakh was an underestimate. This was due to the fact that it was highly improbable that the count of people who self-identified as transgender persons would ever provide an exact number. Over 66 percent of the people that resided in rural regions or villages described themselves as being of a third gender. The census data also revealed that the literacy level in the community is quite low, with just 46 percent of the population being literate. This is in comparison to the overall population, which has a literacy rate of 74 percent. Members of the community have stated, "We are not surprised that the literacy rate is so low among us, because it is very common for transgender people to drop out from school because of the harassment and discrimination we face." The state of Uttar Pradesh had the highest proportion of the sexual minorities/third gender population, which was about 28percent. This was followed by the state of Andhra Pradesh, which had 9percent, Maharashtra, which had 8percent, and Bihar, which had over 6percent. Over three percent of the entire transgender population was found in the state of Rajasthan, while two percent was found in the state of Punjab. The percentage of transgender people who are employed is likewise quite low, coming in at 38 percent when compared to the 46 percent who are employed in the overall population. In conclusion, the article claimed that this is a starting and proud time for sexual minorities/third gender persons because the census could draw out part of the truth and established that the transgender/sexual minority's community does exist and that their literacy rate is very low. This is a beginning and proud moment for sexual minorities/third gender persons because the census could draw out part of the truth and establish these facts. They have also proven the existence of children who transition between genders. It is currently the responsibility of the government to formulate policies to ensure that members of sexual minorities and the transgender community are not subjected to discrimination and that they are granted all of the same rights as children of any other gender.

According to the author Soumya (2014), the most significant obstacle that persons who belong to sexual minorities or who identify as transgender must overcome is the ignorance of their gender identity concerns on the part of medical professionals, who acknowledge only saree-clad patients. Hijras, also known as traditional male-to-female transsexuals, are members of the community who live their lives as transgender individuals. People who identify as transgender asserted that very few medical professionals were aware of the distinctions between homosexuals, intersex, transgender, and transsexual people, and that the majority of practitioners were unable to distinguish between the groups. On the other hand, medical professionals exclusively acknowledge transgender individuals whose gender transition is from female to male. Because of the concern of the stigma that may result, medical personnel and doctors try to avoid any association with people who belong to sexual minorities or who identify as transgender. The fact that a medical doctor with the title "Dr. Devdas" said that "other doctors look down on us if we are sensitive to transgender" demonstrates that there is unquestionably a stigma associated to the community of sexual minorities and transgender individuals working in the field of health care. The author Dinesh C. Sharma (2014) discusses topics such as India's sexual minority/transgender community or Hijra's legal status as a third gender, constitutional protection and Human rights, and affirmative action, including reservation quotas in government jobs, among other topics. This remained challenging for a great number of persons who identify as sexual minorities or as transgender. Under British control, sexual minorities were denied their civil rights and were treated as criminals under the Criminal Tribes Act of 1871. This law was passed in 1871. Even after the ban was abolished in 1952, several municipal laws remained to show a discriminating attitude toward the Hijra population even after it was legal to do so. Hijras continue to be denied a formal identity and fundamental rights such as access to health care services and government jobs; in addition, they are frequently the target of stigma, discrimination, and harassment; and many of them are only able to make a living by begging for alms from shopkeepers, parents of newborn babies, or by dancing at functions, particularly weddings. Hijras continue to be denied a formal identity and fundamental rights such as access to health care services and government jobs. Additionally, some of the Hijras operate in the sex industry. In addition, many members of sexual minorities have voiced their concerns that social exclusion based on identity is preventing them from exercising their rights to property and inheritance, preventing them from receiving health care and welfare benefits, preventing the issuing of identification cards, and limiting their employment opportunities. In conclusion, the author suggests that, as a first step, all sexual minority and transgender populations in the various states will need to be mapped out. This will allow for the appropriate social and economic interventions to be planned, and the author goes on to say that, according to the author's unofficial estimates, the Hijra population in India is approximately one million. At the moment, only one state, Tamil Nadu, has a distinct welfare board for communities of sexual minorities and transgender people, which provides access to government services and benefit programs for such populations. The state of Madhya Pradesh, which recently made their announcement

proposals for a board that is comparable following the decision of the Supreme Court. However, it is a well-known fact that the journey toward achieving equal rights for India's sexual minorities would definitely be an arduous one. The author of Sonu (2015) investigated the cultural and traditional traditions of the Hijra people, who identify as a third gender that is neither men nor women. According to the author, Hijras are cultural performers, religious ascetics, and adhere to their own customs, religious practices, and rituals, in addition to having their very own community activities. According to the author, begging or soliciting alms is not only a profession for Hijras but also a longstanding custom for members of their community. The author goes on to say that Hijras are excluded from the mainstream society and from the common culture of cis gender people. Hijras are involved in the naming ceremony of newly born babies to bless them. They also dance at functions, especially marriage functions.

Their second occupation is commercial sex or sex work. In addition, the author says that Hijras are involved in sex work. Despite this, Hijras have been able to effectively build their own distinct culture. They have their own culture, tradition, kinship, ritual, ceremonies, religion, and so on; they live together, follow their own tradition and customs, and also have a well-established social structure among themselves. Although Hijras are an outlier in society, they have been able to successfully develop their own alternative society. According to Anitha Chettiar (2015), a writer, "The Male to Female (MTF) Transgender in India commonly known as the Hijras are the hardly researched (studied by few), abused, disrespected, and seriously neglected groups in Indian Society." Hijras are a term for transgender people who transition from male to female in India. According to the author of the study, the majority of people who make the decision to convert to Islam come from middle-class and upper-lower class families. The majority of the Hijras who participated in the study reported that they experienced a number of health problems in addition to problems related to harassment, unlawful penalties, sexual abuse, violence, and violation of human rights. When asked who was responsible for the violence and abuse, the majority of respondents named members of the police force, including members of the traffic and railway police.

According to the authors of the study published in 2015 by Nattavudh Powdthavee et al., very little is known about how the differential treatment of sexual minorities/transgender could effect subjective reports of overall well-being. The purpose of this research was to attempt to bridge this knowledge gap. Data from two big polls that give nationally representative samples for two separate countries, namely the United Kingdom and the United States of America. For the purpose of estimating a model of life satisfaction based on simultaneous equations, Australia and the United Kingdom are employed. This model enables for self-reported sexual identity to influence a measure of life satisfaction directly as well as indirectly through a total of seven different factors.

many routes, which are as follows: employment (i), income (ii), marriage and de facto relationships (iii), children (iv), health (v), friendship networks (vi), and education (vii). On the other hand, research has shown that people who identify as lesbian, gay, or bisexual report significantly lower levels of happiness with their life compared to similarly situated heterosexual (cis gender) individuals. This is the outcome of a combination of direct and indirect actions taking place in both of these countries. This article by Kishalaya Mukhopadhaya (2016) examined whether or not heterosexuality and monogamous marriage (with opposite sex) is the only form of relation that existed in the past in India. The author claims that homosexuality (sexual relation with person of same sex) was not a western import. The author examined the Indian ancient Sanskrit texts, as well as medieval Sanskrit texts and medieval Persian/Urdu texts, among other Indian texts. Which clearly show examples of not just the presence of homosexuality practices but also examples of tolerance and celebration of the same, the author goes on to say that sexual minorities and transgender people need to speak up, and they need to reverse the process of being excluded from mainstream society and of being silenced.

According to the author Rashmi Patel (2016), although homosexuality and queer identities may be accepted by more young people in India than ever before, the acceptance of homosexuality and the freedom to openly express their gender choices still remain a constant struggle for them within the boundaries of family, neighborhood, and educational institutions. In urban India, where social media and corporate initiatives have created increasing awareness about LGBT (lesbian, gay, bisexual, and transgender) rights, the situation appears to be more favorable for gay men than for lesbian women or transgender people. On the other hand, families in rural areas of India have their own ways of dealing with LGBT (lesbian, gay, bisexual, and transgender) individuals. In some regions of India, honor killings are arranged in secret, and as a result, the only option for a young gay man to survive is to flee the house in the middle of the night and make his way to another city, despite the fact that he has neither money nor the support of his peers. The author also mentions a recent study that found one of the major factors that results in the stigmatization of LGBT (lesbian, gay, bisexual, and transgender individuals) people is parental reaction towards their homosexuality. The study goes on to conclude that the majority of LGBT people are acceptable to family only if they agree to behave like heterosexuals. The author also mentions that this study was conducted in the United Kingdom.

According to the findings of Cecilia Tomori and colleagues (2016), males who have sexual relations with other men (also known as MSM) continue to be at a significant risk of contracting HIV. MSM's experiences of stigmatization and discrimination, as well as their susceptibility to the risk of HIV infection, may be shaped by culturally particular sexual identities, which include sexual roles, behavior, and appearance. This may further alter MSM's vulnerability to the virus. This qualitative investigation on sexual identity formation, identity practices, and transitions, as well as their implications for HIV prevention, was carried out utilizing focus group discussions (FGDs) and in-depth interviews (IDIs) across a number of different sites in India as part of a multi-site qualitative study. The findings of the study, on the other hand, indicate the varied construction of sexual identities, with MSM who experience larger levels of harassment, violence, gender nonconforming behaviors or appearance reporting greater levels of disapproval and exclusion at large from their families and communities. It was vital in day-to-day life, particularly for married MSMs, to conceal the more feminine elements of their sexual identities. In this study, some of the participants negotiated their identity practices in accordance with cultural and socio-economic pressures. This included adopting identity attributes to satisfy consumer demand in commercial sex work and spending extended periods of time joining communities of Hijras (sometimes referred to as TGs or transgendered women). The participants in this study also noted that some MSMs shift toward more feminine and Hijra or transgender women identities. These transitions were motivated by intersecting desires for feminine gender expression as well as by social isolation and economic marginalization.

According to the author Matthew Stief (2016), sexuality and gender related cultural categories may vary to a notably large stretch. While western cultures have categorized people primarily in terms of their sexual attractions (viz, gay, straight, and bisexual), a lot of cultures differentiate between the groups based on additional issues such as presentation of gender role and position preference in anal sex activity (i.e. insertive/receptive). This study has gathered data on three categories of sexuality and gender related cultural categories. First of all, Hijras are androphilic, which means that they are sexually attracted to adult men. They are also normally sexually responsive in nature, but some of them have had their testicles removed. Hijras reside in fictive familial networks that may be arranged hierarchically. Second, Kothis, like Hijra, are androphilic, meaning that they are normally sexually responsive in nature and relatively more feminine. However, this trait is exhibited by Kothis to a lesser extent than by Hijra since, unlike Hijra, Kothi are never castrated. Some of the participants had the impression that Hijra and Kothi had a mentality that was similar to their own. Additionally, these three groupings were distinguished from one another as being either Hijra solely, Kothi only, or both Hijra and Kothi

as well as Kothi. Thirdly, Panthis are partners of Hijra and Kothi and have a culine insertive quality to their nature. It was discovered that every Hijras and Kothis group possessed an androphilic disposition in its entirety. It was discovered that Panthi men were quite normal in appearance and that their sexual inclinations followed a bisexual pattern. Kothis were found to be less extreme in their female type and to report fewer female gender presentation milestones than Hijras or Hijra/Kothi combined. This was discovered through research. According to the results of the survey, the vast majority of Hijra, Hijra/Kothi, and Kothi respondents all stated that they had not been castrated. In contrast to the way in which they are socially and culturally characterized, very few members of the Panthi group have reported engaging in anal sexual activity, and very few members of the Hijra and Kothi groups have reported engaging in insertive sexual behavior at some point in their lives. This article makes it quite evident that Hijra, Kothi, and Panthi all have sexual characteristics. This article by Anuvinda P, et al. (2016) looked at The Rights of Transgender Persons Bill 2014, which was a private member's bill introduced by Tiruchi Siva, who is a member of the Rajya Sabha. On April 24, 2015, the Rajya Sabha witnessed a historic unanimous passage of the law, making it the first time that this has ever happened. There are two primary reasons why the enactment of the Rights of Transgender Persons Bill ought to be of relevance to the thinking of Indians. It is the only private member's bill that has been passed by either house of Parliament in the past 46 years, and the reasons behind this passing, as well as the reasons behind the non-passage of other private member's bills, need to be studied in great detail. This is the first reason why this measure deserves serious consideration. Nevertheless, as this bill waits to see what will happen to it in the Lok Sabha during the upcoming session of the Parliament, it is vital for us to concentrate our attention on the provisions of the bill that deal with the rights of transgender people. The ideation and drafting of Tiruchi Siva's bill, the bill's passage through the Rajya Sabha, and the uncertain future that the bill faces now have thus far closely reflected the government's apathy while dealing with the significant issue of transgender rights. The bill's birth and life is the ideation and drafting of Tiruchi Siva's bill. In addition, it was hoped that the law would be passed by the Rajya Sabha; nevertheless, it must be confessed that it was never anticipated in accordance with the truth. According to the author, this should not come as a surprise given that they are on the "wrong side of history" and have had 46 years of unsuccessful attempts to enact a bill that was proposed by a private member. The measure was not supported by the might of the government; rather, it was supported by the hopes and prayers of India's long-neglected population of sexual minorities and transgender people. These individuals are visible on the streets but not invisible to the state. The members of the house watched representatives from different parties working together for the bill.

According to a research published by the World Bank in 2016, it is estimated that over 700,000 transgender individuals in India obtain very little or occasionally none of the resources that are available to them. schooling (Education), their families frequently reject them, and transgender persons join marginalized communities where their employment alternatives will be the commercial sex work, singing, dancing, and ritualized begging. schooling (Education) and their families frequently reject them. Lesbians who live openly in a relationship with someone of the same gender in India and who normally exhibit characteristics that are considered to be masculine would be ostracized from their social networks. On the other hand, if their relatives do not kill them by beating them to death — something that may and does happen on a regular basis in rural parts of India — then they will be pushed into marriage. Transgender people may suffer prejudice in the workplace and are often denied access to resources that are already scarce. Because of their femininity (in the case of men), mainstream culture is hostile toward Hijras, Kothiis, gay men, and lesbians, and this hostility often begins at a very young age and escalates into physical aggression. According to the author Akhand Sharma (2018), the trans-women and transgender population in India has a lengthy history that dates back to the beginning of our civilisation. In general, Indian law recognizes transgender women as a third gender; nonetheless, up to this day, these individuals are fighting for their definitive identity, and they are not gaining recognition from the majority of Indian culture. The purpose of this research was to analyze the challenges that the transgender population faces in today's globalized world in terms of social acceptance, education, economic opportunities, political pressure, and a variety of other difficulties. By using the method of case studies, the authors of this study aimed to have a conversation about the sentiments and sensations that transgender people experience, both in the state of Madhya Pradesh and in other states in India. The inventory approach and the experience method were employed as instruments in the study to collect facts, data, and information from members of the transgender community. A series of personal interview sessions have been organized, and various life experiences and incidents of a transgender person's life have been discussed (FGDs) in these sessions. These life experiences and occurrences highlight the challenges that transgender individuals confront in their day-to-day lives. In conclusion, the most important takeaways from this research centered on the initiatives taken by transgender persons in the Indian state of Madhya Pradesh to enhance their reputation and social standing in the hopes of gaining respect and acceptance from the general population. The purpose of the entire study was to bring awareness to the challenges faced by members of the transgender community in today's more interconnected and technologically advanced society.

Studies on the effects of stigma, exclusion, and discrimination on sexual minorities (including their effects on social, economic, legal/political, and health care systems) are included in the second section. This section contains a quick note of the indigenous (researches done in India) and foreign (researches done in other countries) researches, theories, papers, and viewpoints of various researcher academicians, in reference to the discrimination, exclusion, and stigma that is placed on sexual minorities in various scenarios. It is the most accurate and faithful attempt of what has been made in the movement to free sexual minorities/transgender community people in India. However, the article mentions about some unconscious facts such as, till today none of the publications have a lesbian on their editorial board, and the columns in Journals and newspapers are male dominated. This article is about the Gay and Lesbian Movements in India and was published in 1996 by LTE (1996). In addition, the lesbians who served as members of the editorial board of Bombay Dost in 1990 are not currently employed in that capacity any longer. The following is a rundown of the events surrounding this matter: Bombay Dost was initially published by an editorial collective consisting of three gay males and three lesbians. There was no requirement whatsoever for the gay males to collaborate with the women, therefore they did so solely out of a real desire to advance gender justice and equity. As the author points out, there is a willful and purposeful unwillingness to recognise the presence of homosexual behavior in India. Bombay Dost was formed not merely as a platform for gay activism, but primarily to fight concerns linked to unprotected homosexual transmission of HIV infection and STDs. This is because, as the author points out, there is a platform for gay activism. Since the very beginning of the HIV/AIDS crisis, the dispute of the Indian government has been that homosexuality is a result of "western bourgeois decadence." This disagreement has been going on since the very beginning of the HIV/AIDS epidemic. It is possible to link the refusal of the government of West Bengal to agree to sero-surveillance for HIV in the general population back to this refusal to embrace some painful topics relating to sexuality in India. This rejection is the same reason why the government refused to agree to sero-surveillance. In conclusion, not only does this mindset result in the victimization of female sex workers, but it also prevents attention from being focused on the research of the sexual behavior patterns exhibited by the male population.

According to the author Vimal Balasubrahmanyan (1996), even within the circles of those working on development, there is ignorance and prejudice on the issues surrounding homosexuality. Even while some individual activists may be sympathetic, not a single civil liberties organization or group has so far listed LGBT rights as an essential item on their agenda. This is the case even though some of these organizations and groups may be sympathetic. However, the work at hand now is just to bring about the repeal of Section 377 of the Indian Penal Code, which makes homosexuality a criminal crime and nothing more. This is the only thing that needs to be accomplished. The author Alice M. Miller (1999) discusses the idea that activists and other development organizations ought to have the content of progressive, developmental, and transformative rights claims based on their own work in connection to the requirements of a variety of individuals with varying requirements.

placed people of different sexual identities, sexes and genders, races, ages, cultures, ethnicities, nationalities, and other distinctions. According to the author, the final point is that such efforts will force us to verbalize our thoughts on people who are in different situations. This will make a significant contribution to the preservation and promotion of all human rights for persons who are in a variety of diverse situations. In addition, the author places special emphasis on the topic of sexuality, arguing that it is an essential component of every human being. According to the author Arthur S. Leonard (2003), the legal status of lesbian, gay, bisexual, and transgender people (also referred to collectively as sexual/gender minorities) has undergone a partial revolution in the workplaces in America over the past 50 years. This revolution has significantly transformed the status of a sexual/gender minorities, but it is only a partial one because in many parts of America, there is still discrimination against sexual/gender minorities. In addition to this, the implementation of the guarantees of non-discrimination continues to be inconsistent. The author draws a conclusion at the end of the piece, which is that there should be no discrimination based on a person's sexual orientation.

This study, which was conducted by Alok Gupta (2006), aims to investigate the amount and manner in which the condemnation of carnal intercourse against the order of nature under Section 377 of the Indian Penal Code 1860, which classifies homosexuals as criminals, affects the lives of homosexuals. In addition to being a statute regarding anal sex by itself, the Indian Penal Code (IPC) section 377 also relates, in general, to homosexuality. Because there is no distinction in the offense based on whether or not consent was given, some have come to believe that having homosexual intercourse is the same as raping someone and that being homosexual is an inappropriate sexual orientation. The most serious attack on the humanity and dignity of India's sexual and gender minorities was carried out through the Indian Penal Code's Section 377. According to the author, non-discriminatory policies and practices toward sexual and gender minorities will make a direct contribution to restoring the dignity of homosexuals and will make it possible for the sexual and gender minority community movement to emerge from the shadows. According to the author of Prothoma (2007), sexual minorities, also known as non-heterosexuals, are situated on the periphery or fringes of a democracy. This includes those who identify as lesbian, gay, bisexual, or transgender. Sexual minorities are marginalized by the social and political mainstream; they are always cast out of the mainstream by the majority therein (from the heterosexual individuals) they are treated as inferior, incomplete people and also as having unnatural sexual interests, and are considered to be sinners who are wholly unworthy of being in the mainstream.

suffering as a result of some sin that they committed in an earlier incarnation or a previous incarnation. In the case of sexual minorities/non-heterosexuals, sexuality itself is a taboo in the society. The author also says that sexual minorities argue that there is a vast difference between being a minority and becoming a minority or rather being forced to become a minority, and that it is this minoritization and marginalization that they are fighting against. The sexual minorities and non-heterosexuals continue to suffer from no recognition of their existence in the society, not to speak of their The author Christina A. Clark (2007) discussed the idea of human rights as well as how lesbian, gay, bisexual, and transgender (LGBT) issues fit within the framed structure of human rights, legal work, and till now what has been done to secure increased legal rights for LGBT individuals are, as well as a brief overview about the scope of human rights for LGBT individuals in the international community, and further focused on LGBT public policy issues have been discussed. The author concludes by stating that there is a requirement for equality in the human rights to be extended to sexual and gender diversity.

This article by Kenneth H. Mayer and colleagues (2008) discussed the specific needs of LGBT populations (lesbian, gay, bisexual, and transgender collectively referred to as sexual or gender minorities) on the basis of the recent epidemic, clinical systematic study, as well as the difficulties which LGBT population face in obtaining the necessary care and services. LGBT populations include people who identify as lesbian, gay, bisexual, or transgender. In addition, they talked about how experts and staff members working in public health care might improve research techniques, clinical outcomes, and the delivery of necessary services for LGBT individuals. The authors go on to say that homosexuality is not at all a psychiatric illness, but rather that it is a societal and internalized homophobia among heterosexual population that may affect the accessibility of LGBT people towards the necessary care and which cause the mental distress among LGBT people, which in turn might compromise optimal mental health; the study also identified an increase in the rate of sexually transmitted infections among MSMs, and identified the need of awareness for practising medical professionals; the authors of the study also say that homosexuality According to the findings of the study, the collaboration of health care institutions to work together for the welfare of LGBT population and developmental programs for sexual or gender minority populations, as well as the formulation of relevant guidelines and program planning that should run in the present society, is something that should be pursued.

In this report, authored by The Humsafar Trust (2008), an investigation on the major ideas surrounding LGBT (lesbian, gay, bisexual, and transgender) people was carried out. The awareness and actions of LGBT individuals, as well as the stigma and discrimination they face, as well as the indicators for HIV/AIDS prevention among LGBT persons, as well as care and support. A very close examination of the facts that emerged from the studies are as follows: respondents have reflected less stigmatizing attitude, which could be due to the increased exposure to HIV infection related public campaigns and the influence of other print and electronic media; a surprisingly high level of awareness has been detected regarding the transmission and prevention of HIV/AIDS; and respondents have knowledge about HIV/AIDS.

According to the author Jaco Barnard Naude (2008), the equality guarantees in the Constitution of South Africa include sexual orientation as a basis of presumed unfairness discrimination. In South Africa, those who identify as homosexual and who fall outside of the heterosexual hegemony have made significant strides toward achieving freedom as a result of the constitution, which cleared the path for these advancements to occur. According to the author's argument, South Africa has been in the vanguard (like Brazil and India) of the growth of legal developments for gays. This study also tracks and considers these developments, and it argues that any evaluation of the developments for homosexuals should not lose sight of the fact that homosexuals both challenge and acknowledge (even though homosexuals do not necessarily accept or celebrate that) the disciplinary power of the heterosexual (cis gender) hegemony. This study also tracks and considers the developments regarding homosexuals. This section of the study comes to a close with a discussion of the societal obstacles that sexual minorities continue to confront in spite of the changes brought about by the legal system. The author Youngshik D. Bong (2008) investigates the issues that face sexual and gender minorities in Korea, including their struggles against the country's mass media, school system, and legal system. In addition to this, it discusses the most likely direction that homosexual rights movements in Korean society will take in the future and underlines important aspects such as the current situation of sexual and gender minorities. There is no official or reliable statistical data available to measure the actual size of the sexual and gender minority population in Korea, and the government of Korea does not publish any official statistical data regarding the size of the sexual and gender minority population. Additionally, the socio-political visibility of the sexual and gender minority population in Korea still remains very minimal. The idea that there are sexual minorities in Korea is one that is not widely discussed in academic circles; as of the year 2002, there had been just one book produced that was dedicated exclusively to sexual/gender minorities and analyzed how the law treats them.

the status of those who are sexually or gender nonconforming and the instances in which they have been discriminated against. A study titled "Preliminary Study of Human Rights of Sexual Minorities" was issued by the National Human Rights Commission (NHRC) of the Republic of Korea in the year 2005. This report investigates instances of discrimination against sexual/gender minority populations and provides its findings under the title "Preliminary Study of Human Rights of Sexual Minorities." Despite the fact that initially welcoming conditions presented themselves in the LGBT rights movement in Korea, just a few barriers still stand in its way. The fight for the rights of sexual minorities and transgender people in Korea appears to have been successful in improving the social, political, and legal standing of the LGBT population in public life and has now moved on to the next battle front. However, this does not negate the fact that there is still a long way to go. The author concludes by stating that the study of the situation of sexual and gender minorities as well as the homosexual rights movement is a very helpful activity that not only enabled them to grasp the issues themselves, but also provided an inside perspective of the politics that are related to the rights of minorities and the democratic consolidation in Korea. In particular, the author proposes that additional research on this topic is necessary in order to identify and assess the information that helps to define the future trajectory of sexual and gender minority rights in a democratizing Korea. This article by Paul Boycea et al. (2010)

discusses same-sex sexualities, sometimes known as homosexuals, in India. Homosexuals have been portrayed in researches and activism as being socially marginalized and minority groups in the mainstream society. Keeping this in mind, the author of this article takes a critical look at the factors that contribute to the social exclusion of homosexuals. This study points out that, the society is living in the context of post-colonial perspectives on sexuality, and suggests that efforts should be put on to eradicate the marginalization of homosexuals in India. This article has been drawn on the ethnographic researches that have been conducted in different sites. This article intern raises questions about the representation of the queer or same-sex sexual subject in developmental programs, law, and HIV prevention programs.

According to a report published by Human Rights Watch in 2010, sexual and gender minorities in Iran are subject to a disproportionate amount of harassment, discrimination, and abuse at the hands of actors, including members of the actor's family, and also by society as a whole. This is according to an overwhelming majority of the sexual and gender minority individuals that Human Rights Watch interviewed during the course of its investigation. The study also found that the problems that sexual and gender minorities faced were caused by abuse and neglect at their home level. Despite this, sexual and gender minorities in Iran are particularly very much prone to such abuse and neglect because of state law. behavior between people of the same sexual orientation is made illegal, and certain types of same-sex actions can even result in the death penalty. This kind of outrageous remarks or statement which linking to the consensual sexual activity to a disease and simply encourages the discrimination against men who have sex with men (MSMs) Editorial/Ghulam Nabi Azad (2011) this article strongly condemned the statement of a public health officer who said that, the sex between two men is completely unnatural and shouldn't be happen. Nevertheless, the government of India needs to restate its dedication to protecting the rights of each and every one of its citizens, regardless of gender identity, sexual orientation, or sexual behavior that is consented to by the other person. In 2009, India made history by becoming the first country in the world to decriminalize homosexuality through a court ruling. Over the past ten years, India has made significant strides toward protecting the country's sexual and gender minority population. This includes the country's lesbian, homosexual, bisexual, and transgender communities. On the one hand, the government of India has decriminalized homosexuality and taken a huge step toward guaranteeing that people in India are able to express their sexual orientation. On the other hand, the government looks to be engaged in double standards in this situation. despite the fact that its chief public health officer is attempting to cast homosexuality in a negative light. This has the potential to be a significant defeat in the ongoing campaign for sexual rights. If India were to roll back any of the recent progress that it has made toward preserving the rights of sexual and gender minorities, it would be a terrible disgrace. The World Health Organization (WHO) has come around to the idea that it is vital to defend the rights of men who have sex with other males in order to promote safe sexual practices. On the other hand, it has been demonstrated that when men are publicly stigmatized for having sex with other men, they are less likely to seek testing or treatment for HIV/AIDS.

This study was supported by the India HIV/AIDS alliance and was conducted by The Humsafar Trust (2011). This study aimed to understand the impact of the Delhi high court judgement on the lives of members of sexual/gender minorities and to assess the changes as they were perceived and realized by the sexual/gender minority community and stake holders. Additionally, this study was supported by India HIV/AIDS alliance. In the course of this investigation, the data collection took place in three distinct stages before being processed. In the initial step of the process, questionnaires were administered to members of sexual minority communities who have access to the internet (n=75) and to members of sexual minority communities who use cruising sites (n=75). The second stage consisted of conducting interviews with the individuals (n = 10) who had expressed a willingness to talk on video. At the end of the process, the third stage consisted of organizing a consultation with members of the sexual/gender minority group as well as diverse stakeholders. According to the results of the survey, the vast majority of sexual and gender minorities who took part in the research and reported feeling more

sexual and gender minorities have reported feeling more secure in their sexuality and a decline in the amount of violence and harassment they have experienced in recent years. The majority of the participants agreed that there has been a recent increase in visibility in the media; nonetheless, further research indicated that sexual and gender minorities need to claim more social spaces. It was also acknowledged that the challenges confronted by various subpopulations of sexual minorities (individuals who identify as LGBT) are distinct from one another and require individualized forms of intervention.

This article by Antonio Torres-Ruiz (2011) discusses the fight against the HIV/AIDS infection. It is an example of a worldwide struggle for the promotion of sexual health and the protection of human rights for all individuals, particularly the sexual and gender minorities. It provides a challenge to our ability to recognize its impact on the social, political, and economic processes that are taking place. The primary purpose of this piece consists of two parts. First, to highlight the significance of a political and human rights perspective to the analysis of the global response to the pandemic, and for this purpose, the author introduced the concept of policy networks for a better understanding of these dynamics, which can be seen in its second issue; for instance, in the case of Mexico city, the laws of HIV/AIDS policy networks, such as sexual minority activists and public officials, and their actions both internationally and domestically; secondly, to highlight the importance of a political and human rights perspective to the understanding Despite this, major abuses of human rights continue to be committed against those living with HIV/AIDS as well as sexual and gender minorities. This study also intends to investigate the controversy that surrounds globalization and contemporary sexual and gender minority politics in emerging countries, with a particular focus on India as its point of reference. In recent years, India has been witness to an increase in the activism of a number of NGOs and civil society institutions that are working to bring sexual and gender minority groups into mainstream society. Such efforts toward mainstreaming consist of advocacy, which is advocating for the rights of lesbian, gay, bisexual, and transgender groups (LGBTs), campaigning against laws that are discriminating the rights of LGBTs, seeking public petition for withdrawal of such laws, and attempts to normaize sexual orientation and gender identity. In recent years, In contrast, after tracing the history of sexual identity politics, the author of this dissertation evaluated the process of LGBT mobilization in relation to the rise of the HIV/AIDS epidemic and the forces of neoliberal globalization. In addition, the author contends that the twin processes of globalization and the epidemic of HIV/AIDS have greatly influenced the mobilization of sexual and gender minority communities.

This study by Anzu Augustine (2011) examines the experiences of members of the sexual/gender minority community or the transgender community in relation to their citizenship rights. The right to citizenship is connected to a variety of other rights that an individual possesses in respect to their community and society as a whole. Since the beginning of the contemporary democratic era, the numerous dimensions that are connected to citizenship rights have seen significant development. On the other hand, the concept of sexual citizenship did not come into existence until the 1980s, when the third wave of feminism had already cemented its place in the world. Because of its contribution to the diversity as well as the integrity of the concept of citizenship, the idea gained recognition on a global scale. This study's primary focus was on the significance of the sexual citizenship right for the transgender community, which, in the majority of regions of the world, is still regarded as nothing more than a pipe dream by members of this community.

This research was funded by the United Nations Development Program (UNDP), according to The Humsafar Trust (2012). It is a component of a wider investigation that aims to validate the stigma model in India across a variety of contexts. This research effort has tackled the stigma on two separate levels: the individual level and the systemic level. On both of these levels, the demand (men who have sex with other men) and supply (health care professionals) sides would support a holistic understanding of the issue. This, in turn, would be of great assistance in addressing the issues pertaining to access of healthcare services by MSM (men who have sex with men). The sole objectives of the study were to review existing policies and practices within a healthcare (hospital) setup that address issues around stigma and discrimination against MSMs; to know the forms and nature of internalized stigma; to know the perceived obstacles relating to health seeking within the MSM community; and to formulate an advocacy plan. The results of this study suggest that there is a need for work to be done on an institutional level in order to create a balanced atmosphere. Despite this, the training and working with hospitals demonstrate understanding of HIV/AIDS and universal precaution, and many findings have demonstrated a higher level of agreement with the social exclusion of HIV/AIDS positive patients and value judgments against high risk populations (including MSMs). Because there is a significant gap between information and attitude, addressing values and judgments regarding gender, morality, and sexuality ought to be an intrinsic aspect of HIV/AIDS education. The results of the poll have been supported by both the assessment of hospital policy and the observation of patients in hospitals. It is necessary to develop policies on HIV/AIDS prevention and treatment procedures in healthcare settings (hospitals). discrimination on the basis of. Unless there is a balanced and safe environment at the hospital setting, this will act as an obstacle towards HIV/AIDS related health seeking behavior among men who have sex with other men in the hospital setting. These policies should be displayed in the hospital, and the information about these policies should be given to all of the working staff at the healthcare institution.

This study by Abdullah et al. (2012) is qualitative in nature. It consists of in-depth interviews and focus group discussions (FGDs), both of which were carried out in Rawalpindi and Islamabad (both in Pakistan) in the year 2012. According to a number of authors, the Hijra is a particular category of gender role that is practiced in South Asian cultures and involves men doing the duties of women. This group of people is socially excluded by the general community (heterosexuals) in terms of attaining an opportunity for a productive social life. Frequently, this kind of deprivation forces Hijra individuals towards professions like sex work, in pursuit of living (sustenance), which as a result places them as an important piece in the puzzle of an impending generalized HIV/AIDS epidemic in Pakistan. The researchers came to the following conclusion at the end of their investigation: the Hijras had been socially excluded from performing general and regular social functions during various stages of their lives. The Hijras were forced into the high-risk industry of selling commercial sex as a result of the limited employment and educational alternatives available to them. Because the transgender community, also known as Hijras, is socially marginalized in Pakistan, many members of this population have turned to engaging in commercial sexual activity, which puts their lives in grave danger. The authors indicate further that anticipatory steps are very much needed in order to build community-based organizations that are managed and directed by the Hijra community and that address the social isolation and dangerous behaviors of the Hijra population.

According to the writers Sonal Singh et al. (2012), Nepal has been the subject of some reports on abuses of human rights committed against sexual and gender minorities. The primary purpose of the research was to discover a variety of human rights that are both protected by international law and are frequently mentioned by people who identify as belonging to sexual or gender minorities in Kathmandu, Nepal. In the course of this research, three focus group discussions (FGDs) were held in Kathmandu, Nepal, with sexual and gender minority people serving as participants. Trained interviewers led the FGDs. A modified version of the Delphi method was applied in order to collect and rank the definitions of human rights and human rights breaches that were generated by the participants. Data were independently analyzed, and the investigator also performed a cross-check on their work. The participants (n=29) reported that they have been subjected to a variety of abuses of their human rights in a variety of settings, including their homes, educational institutions, places of employment, health care facilities, and public locations

Participants have frequently indicated that they have been subjected to physical assault, mental abuse, and torture. Participants have also not received adequate legal protection. Participants have indicated that gaining access to appropriate legal protection, enhancing family life, and enhancing healthcare services are the most important priority areas for them. However, members of sexual and gender minorities in Kathmandu, Nepal were subjected to a variety of violations of human rights. Therefore, future efforts should be focused on these concerns, which can be of great assistance in integrating sexual and gender minorities into Kathmandu, Nepal's mainstream community.

The author Divya Trivedi (2012) explained the influence that the judicial verdict had on the community of sexual and gender minorities. The judicial decision promised a better sense of self-confidence, which has already moved the community of sexual and gender minorities one step closer to living with dignity. A study that was conducted by the Centre for Health, Law, Ethics and Technology (CHLET) at the Jindal Global Law School discovered that the Delhi High Court's judgment of 2009 on the decriminalisation of consensual gay sex has significantly increased the social acceptance and self-esteem among members of the Lesbian, Gay, Bisexual, Transgender, and Queer (LGBTQ) community. The Delhi High Court's landmark decision of revoking the primitive Section 377 of the Indian Penal Code This has demonstrated to us that mindsets and attitudes are susceptible to change, and that these changes can be brought about by even subtle but progressive amendments to the legislation. It has already taken members of the sexual/gender minority community one step closer to living with dignity, while also holding out the promise of increased self-confidence for the community as a whole. It appears as though the verdict did not have much of an effect, if any at all, on the acceptance shown by the family. The majority of people who responded from the community stated that they would not divulge their identities to their families, and some of the others who had experienced discrimination from their families in the past reiterated this sentiment. Respondent also believed that there should be an environment in which they may live more openly. Author further said that, the laws are needed to change the lives of sexual and gender minorities, one of the respondent said, "I cannot even go home as my sister has to get married." Author further said that, the laws are needed to alter the lives of sexual and gender minorities. When it comes to discrimination, parents can have a significant impact. Author also stated that in order to protect them from discrimination, anti-discrimination laws need to be enacted, and only after that will families be more tolerant.

This study was conducted by Laura H. Thompson and her colleagues (2013) and it focused on the state of Karnataka in India. The findings of this study indicate that stigma and prejudice have become the defining characteristics of sexual and gender minority communities. Kothis, who have been classified as feminine men, have attitudes that are extremely negative regarding the individual's own sexuality in regards to the various aspects of their social life. This article has attempted to restore the voices of those who have been stigmatized and discriminated against by centering its discussion on stigma and discrimination on the subjectivity and moral experiences of Kothis. However, for some of the participants, an awareness of how to deal with the social stigma evolved during the course of the study. This understanding came in the form of an avoidance of public displays of femininity and a cover-up of their sexuality. This mostly reflects the influence that society has on the formation of our subjectivity as well as our conformance to predominately accepted social norms. However, in other contexts—such as those in which same-sex relationships are criminalized or stigmatized—people have been observed to engage in behaviors that are analogous to those used to conceal their sexual identities and adhere to the expectations of heterosexuality held by society.

This essay by Suresh Bada Math et al. (2013) aims to bring to light the violation of fundamental human rights experienced by sexual and gender minorities, as well as the necessity of providing equal opportunities for them and protecting their rights in the same manner as any other citizen who abides by the law. In addition, the authors state that there is a difference in the health care services provided to individuals who belong to sexual minorities in practically every society. For instance, transgender people do not have a distinct ward in any hospital environment, nor do they have any beds dedicated specifically for them. In certain cases, transgender persons are not even permitted to enter hospitals, and those that do not have a designated ward for in-patient care do not have a distinct area designated for their use. Because they are at a high risk for a wide variety of physical and mental diseases, it is imperative that they have access to appropriate medical treatment. The health concerns faced by members of sexual minority groups have been the primary focus of this investigation. The authors go on to state that sexual minorities have a much increased likelihood of contracting sexually transmitted diseases (STDs) such as HIV/AIDS. They are also at an increased risk of being victims of sexual, physical, economic, and emotional violence at the hands of members of the so-called normal community (the community of individuals who identify as cisgender). According to the findings of the study, sexual minorities are subject to health care inequities, which can be eradicated only if medical practitioners are informed about the sexual orientation and gender identity of their patients through reflective, non-judgmental conversation and careful history-taking. According to the author Kaveesher Krishnan (2013), communities of transgender people do not exist in the community, and those who identify as transgender are completely shut out of the mainstream society. The author discusses the major obstacles that must be overcome before the transgender population can be accepted into mainstream society. These obstacles include the non-acceptance of the existence of transgender people in society, the rejection of alternative sexual identities, and the maintenance of family pride.

The author goes on to state that this type of societal exclusion not only causes those who identify as transgender to experience discomfort but also but also maintains the existing disparity and lack of resources. In India, those who identify as transgender belong to one of the most marginalized and vulnerable communities, and their living conditions are often deplorable and insufficient. The author implies that the social, political, and cultural environment has not yet accepted the transgender community's very existence and the fact that they are healthy.

According to the author Trisha Mukherjee (2013), the Government of Bangladesh has made a historic decision when it finally provided its transgender (sexual minorities) citizens with a definite sexual identity by recognizing them as 'Third Sex.' Until this year, the Bangladesh government refrained from identifying them as belonging to any other category except male and female, despite the fact that transgender were given the right to vote in 2008. On their National Identity Card (NID), the information regarding their sexual orientation was left blank. In addition, in order to accomplish the primary goal of the identification System for enhancing access to services IDEA project that was initiated in Bangladesh, this endeavor is currently under way. They are now able to access all processes that require an officially authorized identity because the Election Commission of Bangladesh has included a special column in the NID that marks their sex as 'transgender' with the sign (T). In addition, the transgender population in India continues to be denied legal recognition, which results in them being treated as if they are not citizens of the country. Because of this, they are unable to get the numerous social and economic benefits that are available through the various programs. However, there have been a few recent events in India that are signs of a positive trend wherein the transgender community is progressively getting recognized by the culture. Additionally, beginning in 2005, applications for passports have included a category for "third sex," which is a category for those who identify as having a sexual orientation other than male or female. On their respective registration forms, both the Election Commission of India and the Unique Identification Authority of India (Aadhar) acknowledge the existence of a third gender. On the gender column of the Census taken in 2011, there was additionally a 'other' category. A transgender welfare board has also been established in the state of Tamil Nadu, although the recognition of transgender people by society as having an equal sex status is still a very long way off. However, the matter at hand is no longer limited to the immediate problems that this marginalized minority is facing; rather, the focus has shifted to the legal system, which is examining article 21 of the Indian Constitution, which provides the right to privacy, which includes the ability to express one's gender. The author wonders how much longer it will be before the word "human" may be used to refer to all kinds of people, not only those who are able to classify themselves as either male or female. Editorial Board (2014) The Supreme Court of India has recognized people who identify as transgender as a legally recognized third gender. The judgement of the Supreme Court of India was based on rights given by the Constitution of India as well as legislation from other countries throughout the world.

declared that gender identity and sexual orientation are crucial components of the right to dignity, as well as the right to self-determination and independence. However, in the case involving transgender persons, Section 377 of the Indian Penal Code was mentioned as a means of discrimination against transgender people. Section 377 of the Indian Penal Code prohibits carnal intercourse that goes against the order of nature. The Supreme Court of India did the right thing when it acknowledged the long-standing and varied presence of transgender individuals (sexual minorities) in Indian society. The court went on to name the various traditional categories of people who identify as transgender in India, such as Hijras, Kothis, Aravanis, Shiv-Shakthis, Jogtas, and others. It was very astute of the Supreme Court to make this argument, given that anti-gay rights groups in India have attempted to eradicate the decriminalization of gay sex and transgender identities as degenerate western ideals that are foreign aspects to India's cultural traditions. The Supreme Court's decision to make this point was much wiser. The Supreme Court has ordered the central and state governments to find a solution to the long-standing discrimination that transgender people face. This includes recognizing transgender people as an official minority group, providing transgender individuals with reservations for public jobs and admission to educational institutions, ensuring that transgender individuals are not discriminated against when seeking medical care, and ensuring that official identity documents include a box for a third gender option. The Supreme Court has also decided to hear oral arguments for a petition challenging a judgement that maintains the validity of Section 377 of the Indian Penal Code. This ruling should be overturned since it is past time for Section 377 of the Indian Penal Code to be eliminated.

This is Kumar. The Criminal Tribes Act of 1871 was legislation that was passed by the British government to supervise the actions of the transgender community. This act deemed the entire community of Hijra persons to be inherently criminal. A (2014) this article is about the British law, through the British government; legislation was enacted to supervise the activities of the transgender community. Hijras who seemed to be dressed or decorated like a lady in a public place, as well as those who danced or performed music in a public place, were subject to a penalty under the original version of this Act. It also provided for the registration, surveillance, and control of certain criminal tribes and Hijras. Originally, this Act had also penalized Hijras. Under the Criminal Tribes Act, such Hijra individuals could be arrested without a warrant and given a sentence of imprisonment of up to two years or a fine, or both, depending on the circumstances. The authorities of the area was required to compulsively register the names and addresses of all Hijras who lived there, in addition to the properties that they owned. In spite of the fact that the Criminal Tribes Act had been repealed back in August of 1949, the harm that it had caused had already been done. This study by Tanveer Abbas and colleagues (2014) examines the social adjustment of transgender persons in Pakistan (Chiniot district) and how transgender people are able to survive in this environment. Specifically, the authors focus on how transgender people are able to get employment. Transgender people are a stigmatized and socially ostracized minority in Pakistan. They are frequently connected with activities such as dancing, begging, and prostitution. This study investigates five aspects of transgender life: the social, political, religious, psychological, and individual adjustments of transgender people. According to the findings of the fieldwork that was conducted in Pakistan, the most significant elements that influence the lives of transgender people are age, the members of their families, the structure of their families, and education. This research has demonstrated that family and society can have both positive and bad effects on the lives of transgender individuals. Membership in a transgender community is one of the primary aspects of the lives of many transgender individuals

The author of Kautilya (2015) discusses some of the most significant challenges faced by Mangalamukhis, which is the name given to transgender people in the state of Karnataka, India. Mangalamukhis, in general, do not live with their parents or other close relatives, and they are completely isolated from the social and cultural life of mainstream society. The Mangalamukhis are a poor and property-less people who struggle economically. The disadvantages that the Mangalamukhis confront include the fact that they are frequently expelled from school or college, that they are socially discriminated against, that they are jobless, and that some Mangalamukhis work as brokers in the commercial sex trade, amongst other issues. The author goes on to argue that developing and putting into action a social rehabilitation strategy to assist Mangalamukhis is truly a very difficult and complicated undertaking to undertake. However, although it is highly important to provide housing and other fundamental utilities for Mangalamukhis, this alone will not be sufficient to empower them. There should be a more in-depth discussion in public about this topic because the Mangalamukhis are a unique type of people who are economically disadvantaged and socially marginalized. An employment, social inclusion, and health care-focused plan is absolutely vital for them. As a result, the Indian culture owes them the compassion, sympathy, and love that it can muster. According to a study conducted by Matthew J. Mimiaga and colleagues (2015), men who have sex with other men (also known as "MSM") in India are a hidden and largely less studied population, and their HIV/AIDS prevalence is 17 times higher than that of the general Indian population (which indicates large numbers of heterosexual individuals).

MSM people experience social marginalization, and negative psychosocial conditions occurs concurrently with the HIV/AIDS risk among Indian MSM people. Five focus group discussions (FGD) and nine key informant interviews were done with a total of 55 MSM in Chennai (India), with the goal of better understanding the contextual factors that drive HIV/AIDS risk and informing action for the development of the situation. In relation to their status as gender nonconformists and sexual minorities, participants indicated sources of psychological suffering and low self-worth in the study. the community. These included the pressure from families to marry, the inability of families to accept them, sexual abuse during childhood, and the need to keep their position as a sexual minority a closely guarded secret. The personal evaluations of the participants suggested that self-acceptance may be a significant component that can protect against these psychosocial and HIV/AIDS risk factors. In addition, the findings of the study show out the potential strength of techniques that focus on self-acceptance of one's sexual minority identity to nurture better psychosocial health and also the overall health of Indian MSM. These strategies were found to be effective in supporting health-seeking behavioral adjustments for Indian MSM on an individual level.

According to the author Reshma Elizabeth Thomas (2015), emerging economies like India are undergoing a mobilization of sexual and gender minorities as well as sexual identity politics, which is raising the fundamental questions of human rights, citizenship, tradition, and cultural identity. Additionally, with economic globalization in the developing world, a western hegemonic belief of the Lesbian, Gay, Bisexual, and Transgender (LGBT) identity has been exported to traditional stereotype societies, thereby destroying those societies. This study investigated the consequences of globalization and colonization on the developing world, with specific reference to India. In India, the practice of transgender people has been prevalent throughout history, both in relation to the pre-colonial era and the forces of neoliberal globalization. This topic was investigated in this study. Globalization and colonization are two phenomena that have had a huge impact on the acceptability of LGBT populations in Indian society, while at the same time strengthening the opinion of western historians and academics.

According to a study conducted by Dr. D. Venkatrama Raju (2015), if India were to establish and recognize transgender rights, the country would be in a position to fight against its current HIV/AIDS epidemic in a meaningful way. This would be accomplished by providing the real effect to the human rights of sexual minorities, and it would also serve as a model for other countries around the world to recognize gender-based rights. On the other hand, in order for India to achieve these objectives, it will first need to do rid of its existing discriminatory laws and then pass legislation requiring equal opportunity regardless of a person's sexual orientation or gender. It is necessary to enact formal laws in order to bring about changes that are meaningful. With the assistance of human rights activists and union of members, the formal legislation might very easily be enacted in a manner that is analogous to the most recent ruling of the Supreme Court, in which transgender people are legally recognized as belonging to a third gender.

According to G Karunanithi (2015)'s post, transgender individuals in India frequently have to face a mixture of responses anytime they are in public settings. This is a common experience for transgender people in India. This has forced many of them to reside, for the most part, in places that are designated as slums. An official count places the number of transgender people in India at 4.49 lakh, according to a story that was published in the Times of India on May 30, 2014. Approximately 4.5%, or 22,000, of India's transgender population lives in the state of Tamil Nadu. The transgender community continues to be stigmatized, marginalized, and deprived of political influence, despite the fact that its members make a living by begging and performing sexual services for pay. The majority of Indians appear to have some reservations about recognizing this community since they are preoccupied with the idea of a binary relationship between the sexes and are oblivious to the existence of transgender people. The transgender population has socio-economic challenges as a result of the widespread lack of support from the general public. Because of the precarious position they occupy in society, transgender persons are frequently targets of sexual assault as well as other forms of sexual harassment and exploitation. As a direct consequence of this, individuals are at an extremely high risk of contracting the HIV/AIDS epidemic as well as other sexually transmitted diseases.

According to Aatish Taseer (2016), the provision of the Indian Penal Code known as section 377, which made homosexuality a crime since it was seen to go against the natural order of things, should be repealed. The Indian Penal Code section 377 was partially overturned by the High Court of Delhi in 2009, however it has not yet been completely eliminated. The author continues by stating that Section 377 of the Indian Penal Code (IPC) is a colonial legislation that was enacted in 1860 by British overlords, but India has now adopted it as its own. This statute has been disavowed by the British for quite some time, but what about India? The author believes that everyone should have the right to love one another and hopes that the Supreme Court will reconsider the case against section 377 of the Indian Penal Code and strike down the law. The author Chaitanya Lakkimsetti (2016) examined the influence of multinational advocacy on the legal struggle on sex work and homosexuality in contemporary India. The author says that the significant development for the sexual/gender minorities occurred in 2013, when the Supreme Court of India upheld India's anti-sodomy law (section 377 of the Indian Penal Code), reversing a progressive 2009 judgment by the High Court of New Delhi, to decriminalize adult consensual homosexuality. Nevertheless, the backwards verdict that was handed down in 2013 was issued despite the fact that there was a robust push on a national and international level to get rid of the anti-sodomy law. However, despite the fact that there has been scholarly emphasis directed on sexual minorities and sexual rights in India, with a primary focus on the legal mobilization around the anti-sodomy statute, the class and identity inequalities that exist within the LGBTQ community mean that the techniques for mobilization need to be adapted accordingly.

pitched at a variety of different levels. However, this may be both a limitation and an advantage, as the LGBTQ communities in India have broadened the debate around Section 377 of the Indian Penal Code beyond health and HIV/AIDS to also include discrimination and abuse of human rights, and they have been able to broaden the conversation around sexuality. This has the potential to be both a limitation and an advantage. This paper by Shilpa Khatri Babbar (2016) is an attempt to shift the focus of social justice, from distribution to a dignified recognition. It does so primarily with reference to the injustices associated with gender and sexuality, both of which are seen by the author as socio-cultural and are seen to have their roots in social patterns of interpretation, representation, and communication. The author believes that this shift is necessary in order to address the injustices associated with gender and sexuality. In addition, the primary purpose of this research was to shed light on the situation of transgender people in India. This was done against the backdrop of the Indian legal system having acknowledged the absurdity of transgender people existing, and despite being sympathetic to transgender people to the point of even granting them recognition, the legal system has been unable to ensure that transgender people can live dignified lives.

According to the author Virginie Dutoya (2016), academic and research writing on homosexual's lives, sexualities, and identifications has developed considerably in India over the past 20 years. This is in a context where Lesbian, Gay, Bisexual, Transgender, and Queer (LGBTQ) politics have become more visible in the public space. When it comes to issues of sexuality and gender, researchers are frequently activists, and scholarship is highly political. However, social scientists contribute in the development of social categories that might be mobilized in the public arena by documenting homosexual lives, activities, and groups. In particular, this aspect of their work focuses on documenting homosexual communities. According to the information provided in this article, social scientists are currently involved in the process of representation with regard to LGBTQ individuals and groups. However, this process is not without difficulties since there is a profound refusal between the production of an object of study that is argued about and the promotion of a political subject who can speak for him or herself. There is a deep refusal between the making of an object of study that is debated about and the promotion of a political subject who can speak for him or herself.

M.H. According to the findings of a study by Hebbal (2018), transgender persons are frequently confronted with a variety of obstacles, including unfairness, deprivation, and discriminatory inclinations in today's society. This study was carried out to gain a better understanding of the socioeconomic status, health state, and abuses of human rights experienced by transgender individuals. A study found that transgender persons live below the poverty level in all aspects. Transgender people are vulnerable to a variety of disadvantages, including threats to their health, violations of their human rights, and economic discrimination.

limits and restrictions. They have been the most economically marginalized, as well as the most economically, socially, and educationally backward sector of the society. People who identify as transgender can suffer from poor health and a variety of other health-related issues. These individuals are also deprived of the municipal amenities and fundamental medical care facilities that are available to them. People who identify as transgender have also mentioned having to live on the streets at some point in their lives. A study recommended that the government and non-governmental organizations (NGOs) take action to integrate the transgender people into society by ensuring that they have access to appropriate levels of healthcare, education, employment, and safety. According to the findings of the research conducted by Catherine Meads and colleagues (2019), the authors of the study discovered that sexual minority people have poorer health and disproportionately higher behavioral hazards to their health than heterosexual people. In this study, a mixed-methods systematic review was used to analyze recent studies on the health experiences of persons who identify as belonging to a sexual minority in the United Kingdom. The analysis was carried out using narrative theme description and synthesis. Sexual minorities reported more unfavorable health experiences, which may have a detrimental affect on access to services as well as the quality of health outcomes. The findings of the study highlighted substantial difficulties that are encountered by sexual minorities. These barriers include hetero-normative beliefs, assumptions, and experiences of negative responses to coming out; ignorance and discrimination from healthcare professionals; and impediments to reporting concerns or complaints. The study also underlined the necessity for specific and consistent education training for healthcare personnel on the challenges that affect sexual minorities, as well as the necessity for stronger application of non-discrimination legislation in healthcare settings.

The Existing Knowledge Gap

The available literature review on sexual minorities and all aspects related to the life of sexual minorities shows that many researchers from anthropology, sociology, economics, human rights, social work, human development, and health care, among other fields, have consistently observed that sexual minorities are highly vulnerable in all aspects. This is the conclusion drawn from the review of the available literature on sexual minorities and all aspects related to the life of sexual minorities. Despite the many changes in laws, the question that needs to be addressed is whether or not sexual minorities, along with other people in the community, are able to encounter safe and positive spaces where people do not hold a stigmatized attitude towards sexual minorities on the basis of their sexual orientation or gender identity is still a question. They are not generally accepted in societies that span nations, and they are the disadvantaged groups in society.

to the culture we live in. Studies that were discussed in the literature section focused solely on topics such as ways of life, cultures and traditions, issues related to HIV/AIDS, social and legal discrimination, the current status of sexual minorities in various locations, human rights violations and atrocities, psychological aspects, support systems that are available, gender identity of sexual minorities, etc. Very few studies have been carried out up until this point that are capable of measuring the perception of sexual minorities with regard to the social exclusion and discrimination that they have personally undergone and are now enduring. As a result, the purpose of this study was to investigate the perspectives held by members of sexual minorities regarding the social exclusion they have endured throughout their lives.

The Final Thoughts.

The preceding debate on literature evaluations are from India and other nations, and they have addressed practically all aspects of the life of sexual minorities in a variety of contexts. Understanding the various problems that are related with sexual minorities and locating the research gaps that exist in these studies has been made easier thanks to the reviews that have been offered in this section. The current study, on the other hand, discovered a gap in the existing research and set out to investigate sexual minorities' perceptions of the social exclusion they have faced in the past and continue to face in their lives.

Summary

The persistent and harmful practice of discrimination on the grounds of caste, religion, place of residence, culture, gender, or sexuality can have the consequence of excluding people from society. These kinds of discriminatory practices might give rise to exclusive practices. These processes of exclusion can take on a variety of forms; social and cultural exclusion can take the form of discrimination along a number of dimensions, including gender, ethnicity, and age. This discrimination lessens the opportunities for individuals who belong to these groups to gain access to social services and restricts their ability to participate in the labor market. The denial of citizenship rights such as the right to organize and participate in politics, as well as personal safety, the rule of law, freedom of expression, and equal opportunity, can be considered a kind of political exclusion. Lack of access to employment, credit and other kinds of capital assets, lack of support from financial institutions, and other similar factors can all be considered types of economic exclusion. Exclusion from health treatment can occur for a variety of reasons, including prejudice in the healthcare industry, carelessness in health systems, etc. These varied exclusions are developing as a consequence of the various causes. These factors, which have a significant impact on the lives of sexual minorities, can be investigated from a number of different points of view. The current study did have an objective, which was to investigate the Causes of social exclusion as perceived by the respondents. In order to achieve this objective, the researcher interviewed only respondents from the community of sexual minorities, and as a result, the data on the causes of social exclusion only reflect what community members think about possible causes for such exclusion. We give both our findings and our comments on the factors that contribute to social isolation here;

Fear of Sexual Minorities (Homophobia): 66.5% of respondents claimed that Homophobia is the primary reason for their exclusion in society; Phobia about sexual minorities or transgender by the dominant heterosexual (cis gender) population is what leads to marginalization. Homophobia is the fear of homosexuals and other sexual minorities. The majority of people in society are heterosexual, and the majority of those people have an odd phobia, and that fear is the primary reason that sexual minorities are excluded from society. This serves as an alarm that awakens the mainstream from their slumber of familiarity at a time when the Hijra community is gradually beginning to ask for its rights. In today's society, the Hijra community is gradually beginning to assert itself. Leaving aside oppression and marginalization, there have been reports of different forms of violence that are fundamentally motivated by homophobic inclinations. According to the viewpoint of a Hijra college student who took part in the survey, a portion of mainstream society may claim that they are progressive and wish to embrace people from underprivileged parts of society as well, but in most cases, this assertion is not genuine and is merely a pretense to show off their faux inclusive character. Even though the majority of his contemporaries are aware of his sexual identity and act as though they accept it, he claims that deep down they are homophobic, which is evident from the way in which they behave and the way in which they think. percent of heterosexual or cisgender people in dominant societies believe that a lack of understanding about sexual minority communities is the primary factor contributing to the marginalization of sexual minorities in society. The fact that there is very little information regarding what the LGBT community genuinely entails is the primary driver behind the existence of this cause. The absence of visibility has meant that all of the members of the community continue to remain concealed, and that the reality of their situation is never revealed to the general public. Aversion is frequently caused by a lack of understanding, which in turn is caused by a decreased representation of the topic in social, political, and cultural spheres, which is again caused by oppression, marginalization, and stigmatization. As a result, it is possible to refer to it as a viscous cycle. A handful of the respondents mentioned that they would like to see more contact at all levels, and there is an increase in understanding coming from the mainstream. This indicates that there has been some progress.

The majority of respondents (49.7 percent) stated that the stigma and taboo that is associated with the sexual minority population is the primary factor that contributes to their exclusion from society. To stigmatize someone or something implies to label them or it as something that should be avoided at all costs. A social stigma is a severe form of social criticism that can be attached to views or characteristics that go against the cultural standards that are common in a culture. Marginalization is a common consequence of stigmatization. They are not living with their families because either the family has rejected them or they are not going back as it would be stigmatizing for the families to have a Hijra in the family. Additionally, it has been shown that public stigmatization of sexual minorities leads to fewer of them seeking testing or treatment for HIV/AIDS. This is a problem because HIV/AIDS is the leading cause of death among sexual minorities. Even medical professionals want to avoid any association with transgender patients because they are afraid of the stigma that may result. "In a hospital other doctors look down on you if you are sensitive to transgender there's definitely a stigma attached" (Boundless), members of the sexual minority community are subject to discrimination and stigma in the mainstream culture due to their sexual orientation. The community is avoided, and very few people in the society even know it exists. The community's visibility in the larger society is extremely low. As a consequence of this, they are excluded from society, where they face scorn and marginalization at the hands of the majority heterosexual population.

Cultural Difference: Among the respondents, 48.4 percent agreed that the primary reason for the sexual minority community's exclusion from mainstream heterosexual culture is the cultural difference between them and the heterosexual majority. Even though the practice of homosexuality has been present in traditional civilizations since the beginning of time, sexual identity has never been a topic of political contention in any of these societies until very recently. In a similar vein, in India, even though it was a part of the culture in ancient times, as shown by old literature, architecture, and other historical evidences, things have taken a radically different turn ever since the colonial periods. Present day The culture of mainstream heterosexuals places sexual minorities on the outside of its circle as unacceptable. The rituals, practices, and traditions of sexual minority communities are completely distinct from those of the mainstream heterosexual community. 5. *Non-human creatures:* According to 43.2% of respondents, cis gender people believe sexual minorities to be non-human beings. This view held by cis gender people is the primary factor that contributes to sexual minorities' marginalization from society. Sexual minorities or communities of people who identify as third gender have always been present in virtually every region of the world. They continue to be a neglected part of society, which results in them being subjected to atrocities and experiencing a variety of types of ill treatment in the context of the *family, the neighborhood, the community, and society as a whole. They are unable to live a social life worthy of their dignity as a result of the divergent perceptions and attitudes held toward them by the members of the society who identify as cisgender. In today's society, those who belong to sexual minorities are frequently viewed as though they are not even human. Hijra Occupation: 72.3% of respondents claimed that the occupation (Hijra Occupation) that they do is the primary cause of their isolation in society. This was found to be the case in the majority of cases. The ancient scripture known as 'Kama Surtra' was written in the fourth century and details the lifestyles and occupations of sexual minorities. It lists the jobs that are approved for transgender people, such as flower sellers, masseurs, and hairdressers, amongst others. However, in today's society, sexual minorities are still involved in occupations such as dancing, despite the many changes that have taken place over time in regards to the jobs held by members of this group. Singing, Begging, (Basti), Blessing (Badhayi), and Sex Work — this form of activity made them stand out from the other heterosexual individuals, which in turn contributed to the isolation of sexual minorities.*

Based on the analysis and interpretation of the data, as well as the primary conclusions of the study, it was determined that there is, in fact, exclusion in the mainstream society for persons who belong to sexual minority groups. This is essentially the result of social structures, the upkeep of those institutions, and certain instances of homophobia that are inherently present in the society. These instances of homophobia are

SUMMARY 199

there for a variety of causes, which were discussed in earlier chapters. The circumstance can be improved, and the levels of exclusion can be reduced, by adhering to certain procedures. To begin, there is advocacy, which is a strategy that is used in social work and is one of the methods that may be utilized to effectively build up a public opinion regarding the subject. There has been a recent rise in the number of advocates calling for equal rights for the community of sexual minorities, and this has been accomplished through Through advocacy, the vast majority of the challenges faced by sexual minorities can be overcome. However, such a shift cannot take place in a single day; rather, it calls for persistent efforts. • Recently, there has been an increase in the visibility of the sexual minority community, and certain urban metros have begun organizing pride marches for the LGBT community, which are attracting an increasing number of people each year. As a result of this increase in visibility, the majority of cis gender people in society are rethinking their attitudes toward the members of the sexually marginalized groups, and many respondents spoke of such changes and expressed their hope that the situation would improve. Through the use of the community organization approach of social work, events such as pride marches can be planned and organized. One of the primary areas that social work interventions should work on is to build a stronger collaboration between various groups working on various elements of sexual minority issues, including organizations working on sexual minority issues. This should be one of the primary areas that social work interventions focus on. It is important for organizations to work together and make a concerted effort to demand their rights as a group; doing so will be the most productive approach to integrate sexual minorities into mainstream society. They should begin to ask for their rights collectively if the LGBT community has any hope of seeing a better world in the future, one in which they are not excluded from participation on the basis of their sexual identity. Remember that in a democracy, strength comes from having a large population. Another suggestion made by the researcher is that all of the efforts to better the sexual minority population should continue to be focused mostly in urban areas. Because there is so little effort put into helping the people living in rural areas, there has been a significant increase in the number of people moving to urban areas. This group absolutely must have some kind of support structure in the locations where they live. Therefore, there has to be a greater level of awareness regarding these topics, which would foster an environment of understanding among the general populace. A certain degree of exclusion for this community was also observed in the health care elements; hence, the researcher advises that the Government Health Department should assume the obligation for providing free health facilities for sexual health concerns. Major hospitals should have a separate department that would provide the medical, surgical, psychological, and counselling assistance for sexual minorities. In this regard, the government may establish counselling centers at taluka level. The health care providers should be sensitized thoroughly about the issues and problems of the LGBT population. Because health is the basic right of every individual, denial of treatment and uncomfortable behavior should be considered as an offense. A recent study found that the majority of the challenges faced by sexual minorities are attributable to the incorrect perception and lack of proper knowledge of the cis gender population regarding LGBT issues. This, in turn, leads to the exclusion and discrimination of the LGBT community. In order to eradicate this type of gender demarcation, it will take some time and ongoing efforts. It is possible to accomplish this goal through the educational system, the media, non-governmental organizations (NGOs), and the government by implementing a variety of programs, such as incorporating gender-sensitive topics into the curriculum, raising awareness about gender issues through the media, and organizing community-based initiatives by NGOs.

Non-governmental organizations and other community-based organizations should help sexual minority population form an association that can represent the community and should promote leadership among sexual minorities. This will most certainly assist sexual minorities in becoming more organized within the state. Additionally, a community center should be opened in all of the major cities for sexual minority population to meet and as a venue for discussion and other activities. Additionally, non-governmental organizations should help sexual minority population form an association that can represent the community and should promote leadership among sexual minorities.

The interventions of NGOs have offered some benefits for sexual minorities, such as counseling services, financial assistance, and inspiration to lead a life, and certain NGOs have become the voices of the communities that are sexual minorities. However, non-governmental organizations (NGOs) that work with sexual minorities should also provide education, healthcare, human rights, and other developmental services to sexual minorities. As a result, NGOs working with sexual minorities should be recognized by the government and financed by large firms as part of their corporate social responsibility programs. Another finding of the study was that, despite the increasing number of educated people in our country and growing exposure to the mass media, society as a whole still carries a lot of misconceptions and incorrect information on sexual minority population; Here, the role of mass media is much important, mass media should make programs on the life of sexual minorities which would give correct information insight about the plight of these people. • Another finding of the study was that, despite the increasing number of educated people in our country and growing exposure Universities and other educational institutions should conduct sensitization workshops or seminars on the rights and life of sexual minorities to create an awareness in the general public and the role of medial is very crucial in this regard, media should work on behalf of marginalized population (such as sexual minorities), media should create awareness among people and make programs on the lives of sexual minorities in helping them to get their rights and dignity;

media should work on behalf of marginalized population (such as sexual minorities); and media should work on behalf of marginalized population (The findings of the study indicate that there is, in fact, a form of social isolation for persons who belong to sexual minorities in mainstream society, and that this has resulted in a variety of psychological issues among members of the sexual minority population. Therefore, as a component of social work activity, free counseling services should be made available to members of the LGBT community through primary health centers in rural regions, as well as through government hospitals and non-governmental organizations in metropolitan areas. This should be done by social workers who have been trained and made aware of LGBT issues. A variety of approaches, such as "outreach programs for the family" and "sensitization programs for the public," among others, should be utilized by social workers in order to raise awareness regarding sexual minorities among family members as well as the general public. A study showed that despite the fact that sexual minorities have access to education, they are lacking in knowledge and awareness about human rights, health issues, government schemes, and other topics. Additionally, the issues of access to legal rights, inheritance of property, legal adoption of child, proper success to public place, and other topics should be addressed by the government. Additionally, a small number of sexual minorities have reported atrocities committed by police officers; consequently, it is necessary to direct the police department to act in response to these allegations. In addition to that, it is essential to raise awareness on these matters among sexual minority groups.

A study found that the government pays little attention to the sexual minority community. This led to a number of problems, including a lack of proper identity, denial of equality, no political representation, no opportunities for employment, no reservations, no opportunities for employment, no political representation, lack of proper identity, and denial of equality. The majority of people who participated in the study stated that they do not even have access to any kind of government facilities. As a result, it is recommended that the government take the appropriate steps to eliminate the une The government ought to set up a commission at the national level to handle matters of this nature and to strive toward the protection and empowerment of those involved. A number of respondents voiced the desire for sexual minority communities to have access to separate public restrooms; the government should build separate public restrooms for sexual minorities in large cities with high populations of sexual minorities; in addition, the government should offer financial assistance, identification cards that accurately reflect their gender, free education and health care for sexual minority communities, freedom for sexual minority communities to observe their own cultural and spiritual values, and the ability to use those facilities. etc.——

The findings of the survey suggest that the majority of respondents do not have Driving license PAN cards, and some respondents do not have Aadhar cards; this demonstrates the shortage of identification documents in the country. identity proofs among sexual minorities and among the respondents who have the identity cards the gender 'Male' has been given in their various identity cards given by the government to the sexual minority community. This was found both in the sexual minority community and among the respondents who have the identity cards. This demonstrates that the government does not have a correct identity for such a community; this problem should be rectified, and the government should also build a separate database of sexual minorities to help deal with the issues and requirements of sexual minorities. Sexual minorities as a collective group are currently living in a separate community that is ignored by the majority of society. The findings of the study indicate that the government does not have a proper identity for such a population. Furthermore, researchers have discovered that it is difficult to find sexual minorities in the society, as they are a hidden community within the society and there is a lack of proper population data or a census of the members of this community. Because people of diverse sexual orientations are not counted separately in the national census, the exact number of people who identify in this way is unknown. In light of this, research argues that they should be accorded the attention they deserve, and the government should make the identification and counting of members of sexual minority communities its top priority. The findings of the study indicate that a greater proportion of respondents are engaged in hijra occupations such as dancing, singing, *begging (Basti), blessing (Badhayi), and prostitution; members of the sexual minority population who make a living by dancing, singing, and begging may be resistant to any form of work that requires physical labor; in addition, sexual minorities who are involved in prostitution need to be rehabilitated because the act of prostitution is associated with a great deal of Therefore, the social and vocational rehabilitation of sexual minorities should be a priority for the government's agenda. Sexual minorities should be provided with appropriate vocational education, training, and rehabilitation, and they should also be rehabilitated in all aspects of society, including work, housing, and health care.*

The research revealed that the majority of the people who participated in the survey took up the Hijra Occupation because there were few alternative employment opportunities available to them. The participants in the study all agreed on one point: they want to be able to support themselves financially, without having to rely on the generosity of others, and they want their communities to have more opportunities for employment. The state should make basic vocational job options available, and there should also be reservations for members of sexual minority populations in higher education, employment (in both the public and commercial sectors), and other sectors and programmes. The findings of the study showed that respondents had feelings of insecurity and harassment whenever they went to public places in the city for the purpose of engaging in fun and leisure activities. As a result, it is essential to raise knowledge among the general population in order to make it possible for members of sexual minorities to freely visit public places including parks, movie theaters, banks, and shops without the fear of being harassed. There is a pressing need to develop a national policy for sexual minorities at this juncture. The most backward and marginalized members of society are those who belong to sexual minorities. It has been discovered that they are even denied the fundamental rights and opportunities guaranteed to them by their constitution. As a result, both the central government and all state governments should create A State Policy specifically for sexual minorities and should assure enough budgetary allocation for the purpose of uplifting and developing sexual minority population in their respective states. In every single one of the plans and decisions pertaining to the policies and programs for sexual minorities, representatives of the communities that are comprised of sexual minorities ought to be included in the decision-making processes. Sexual minorities need to be granted their basic rights and equitable chances, both of which could help them become more self-reliant. Because the majority of people who participated in the study were uninformed of the judicial decisions that have been handed down regarding sexual minorities, the state ought to ensure that all transgender people are aware of all of the judgements that have been handed down by the courts from time to time. The participants expressed a need for awareness programs that would disseminate knowledge about the sexual minority population in the society. The goal of these programs would be to educate heterosexuals in the society and dispel incorrect perceptions about the sexual minority community, which contribute to prejudice and exclusion. Everyone who identifies as a member of a sexual minority craves respect from mainstream society.

Conclusion

In 1956, at a meeting of the American Psychological Association, a psychologist by the name of Dr. Evelyn Hooker was the first person to identify sexual minorities as normal. She did so at that time. (Anasuya Ray) Despite the fact that there is historical evidence to suggest that homosexuality was actually a component of ancient culture across the globe, it is socially unacceptable in the majority of countries on the planet. Sadly, this pattern has not yet reversed itself, and even in modern times, the vast majority of state governments and communities consider homosexuality to be an aberration that should not be tolerated. The Hijra people are excluded from contemporary society in India despite the country's long history of sexual minorities, which is the reason why modern society excludes them. On the other hand, the Hijra people are subjected to a variety of inconvenient aspects, injustices, deprivations, and discriminatory inclinations in modern society. The humiliation of sexual minorities, harassment of sexual minorities, discrimination of sexual minorities, and violence against sexual minorities, together with the denial of legal rights and equal safeguards, are all ultimately rejections of recognition. Without a doubt, members of sexual minori-

ties are also subjected to severe and numerous types of cultural and socioeconomic oppression. The Hijra people are subjected to a number of socioeconomic disadvantages, abuses of human rights, and economic restrictions. They have traditionally been among the least advantaged in terms of educational attainment and economic standing in our society. In addition to this, they face health-related challenges as victims. In addition to this, they are denied access to the civic amenities and fundamental medical facilities that are rightfully theirs. A number of the respondents mentioned that they have been homeless at some point in their lives. People who identify as members of sexual minorities face barriers in society that make it difficult for them to fully access and appreciate the rights that are guaranteed to them as citizens. The idea that only "normal" people should be entitled to full rights of citizenship can manifest itself in discriminatory practices within the legal system and within the social institutions of a society.

However, TGs have had the right to vote since 2009, were recognized in the census in 2011, and were given a separate category as 'others' in the Aadhar card by the Unique Identification Authority of India in 2009. The Indian government made a proposal for a benefit program in December 2014 with the intention of assisting families in providing support for transgender youngsters. Additionally, there is talk of instituting a monthly stipend for transgender children who are enrolled in secondary schools, as well as aid for the development of skills and a pension for transgender adults aged 40 to 60. The plans *were established with the intention of aiding transgender persons in obtaining an education and skills that they may utilize to obtain job and to live their life with dignity. In 2014, the Supreme Court of India issued a landmark verdict in the case of NALSA vs. Union of India, in which it acknowledged transgender individuals as belonging to a "third gender." In addition to the other suggestions, the highest court requested that all states include Hijras within their social welfare systems. projects, and there is also the request that they be included in the OBC category so that they can take advantage of the benefits offered by various programmes run by the government. The government should take measures to integrate members of sexual minority communities into society as a whole by ensuring that these communities have access to acceptable levels of medical care, education, economic opportunities, and basic comforts. The current research is an attempt to investigate the problem of social exclusion experienced by sexual minorities in the Dharwad area of the state of Karnataka. The research was carried out in order to accomplish a number of goals, including gaining a better understanding of socio-demographic status and gender issues, as well as the perceptions of the respondents regarding the social exclusion that they had personally encountered and the factors that were thought to be responsible for such exclusion. As a result, one can reach the conclusion that an exhaustive effort was made in this study to investigate the social isolation experienced by sexual minority communities. A study looked into the many kinds of exclusion, as well as the factors that contribute to it. This research, on the other hand, does not go very deeply into the complexity of identities that are present within the sexual minority community itself; rather, it investigates different types of social segregation and exclusion and attempts to trace the reasons for these phenomena based on the respondent's view of them. Culture and social influences are the primary contributors to the formation of a minority identity. The research focuses on those different influences in its deliberations. People are separated from one another and forced to move further apart because the mainstream labels and categorizes as abnormal any love or form of expression that deviates from the norm. Following an examination of the primary data and the results of the research, the investigator is able to draw the following conclusion: Social exclusion refers to the absence of or denial of rights, resources, goods, and services, as well as the inability to participate in the normal relationships and activities, which are available to the majority of people in a society, whether in the social, economic, political, or cultural arenas. If individuals are going to flourish and reach their full potential, their communities must provide them with opportunities to fully engage in the life of the community. But there are some groups in society that are routinely denied access to opportunities that are available to other people because they are subjected to discrimination on the basis of their racial or religious background, gender, caste, age, handicap, or some other aspect of their social identity. Even though all of the respondents have been subjected to at least one form of exclusion, they themselves do not know what could be the possible way out of this situation and leading them to the mainstream of the society. This is due to the fact that the dominant heterosexual people in the society have closed their minds to the sexual minority community and excluded them from their lives. However, researchers are holding out hope that these issues will be resolved; that the social inclusion of sexual minorities will commence; and that one day, perhaps in the distant future, members of communities of sexual minorities would be able to coexist with their heterosexual peers in a manner that is respectful and dignified.*

Printed in the USA
CPSIA information can be obtained
at www.ICGtesting.com
LVHW091810241023
761966LV00002B/322